THE CANCER CONUNDRUM

THE CANCER CONUNDRUM

STOP DYING—START LIVING

RICK HILL

iUniverse, Inc.
Bloomington

The Cancer Conundrum
Stop Dying—Start Living

iUniverse books may be ordered through booksellers or by contacting:

iUniverse
1663 Liberty Drive
Bloomington, IN 47403
www.iuniverse.com
1-800-Authors (1-800-288-4677)

ISBN: 978-1-4759-1534-1 (sc)
ISBN: 978-1-4759-1536-5 (hc)
ISBN: 978-1-4759-1535-8 (ebk)

Printed in the United States of America

iUniverse rev. date: 05/17/2012

To Dr. Ernesto Contreras R., and to his son,
Dr. Francisco Contreras,
whose courage has provided hope to thousands
of desperate people.

CONTENTS

PREFACE

(Written originally for *Too Young to Die* on September 5, 1991)

Rick Hill came to see me for the first time on a busy morning in the fall of 1974, when he was looking for an alternative in the treatment of his cancer. A few weeks earlier, he had undergone surgery at the Mayo Clinic, where they diagnosed a very aggressive embryonal cell carcinoma. The doctors urged him to start a strong chemotherapy protocol if he wanted to have a good chance of survival. The surgeon and the oncologist were shocked when Rick refused the chemotherapy. When Rick told them he wanted to try a nontoxic program, they warned him that his decision was foolish and predicted fatal consequences.

Rick, unafraid, came to consult me. When I looked over his medical records, my orthodox background told me that this young man was playing with fire. He was such a joyful, positive thinker, and his optimism was so contagious, that I did not hesitate to give him complete freedom of choice. I recommended a completely nontoxic, nonaggressive program. We both prayed that God's will would be done and felt assured that all would be right. And it surely was. He has been in complete remission since 1974!

I am sure that orthodox practitioners would consider Rick's wonderful response to natural methods to be just another case of spontaneous remission, totally anecdotal, with no statistical significance. Well-documented spontaneous remissions (occurring for no apparent reason) or regressions in cancer are extremely rare: one in every eighty thousand or a hundred thousand cases. (Author's note: log on to http:// www.oasisofhope.com to see current statistics.) This is the official criterion. However, after spending twenty-five years treating cancer with nontoxic and natural programs, I have quite different statistics. In strictly orthodox media, the nonconventional methods are still considered a hoax, or at least totally ineffective, producing just a placebo effect. But then why do we see spontaneous remissions so frequently?

My explanation, not only in Rick's case but also in thousands of other cases, is simple. Medicine practiced as a pure science, working only in the biological area, will always have many problems treating cancer, and spontaneous regressions will continue to be the exception. But medicine practiced as an art/science, giving due importance to natural methods and to the care of the cancer patients' psychological and spiritual areas, will produce much better results, and so-called spontaneous regressions will occur more frequently.

Orthodox doctors use the term "spontaneous" because they can't find a reasonable explanation for those regressions in which, scientifically speaking, nothing has been done to the patients. But we know now that good nutrition, vitamins, nontoxic antitumor agents, positive thinking, and a good spiritual attitude are extremely helpful and can no longer be considered placebos. They will soon constitute a basic part of the multidisciplinary management of cancer.

I believe it is time to forget old misunderstandings and rivalries between the conventional and nonconventional doctors for the sake of real progress in the treatment of cancer. I hope that this book will give readers a wider perspective and a better understanding of how to prevent and treat malignant disease. Rick Hill's personal experience will be a great inspiration and an example for doctors and lay people of what oncology will be in the near future: less aggressive, more human, and, best of all, more effective. Life is our most precious gift from God, and we must do our best to make it abundant and productive. I thank God for Rick's life and testimony.

Respectfully yours,

Dr. Ernesto Contreras R., MD
Tijuana, Mexico

ACKNOWLEDGMENTS

In the many years since I have regained my health, countless people have helped me. There is, of course, the entire Contreras family, who have worked tirelessly to save lives. Even though the doctors at the Mayo Clinic were working with a different game plan, they were no less dedicated to making a difference for the people they served. The late, great Lester Bardwell gave me lots of love and time to help get me through this. Barb Hill jumped in with both feet and went on the diet with me, making things much easier. The faithful people of the First Baptist Church in New Ulm, Minnesota, not only prayed for me but gave generously to send me to the Oasis of Hope Hospital in Tijuana, Mexico. My brother Roger edited at least three versions of this book over the years and lived through all of this with me. For this version, my gratitude goes to Jane and Mark Hansen. Mark was smart enough to marry Jane, and Jane was smart enough to do the final edit. Last but not least, *Soldier* Burford was our lifeline for the first week in Tijuana.

PART ONE

DETROIT, MICHIGAN 1966

"E" IS FOR EUNUCH

Detroit was a magical place in the fifties and sixties. Financially, it was one of the focal points of the entire planet; the auto industry held a prominent place in the postindustrial US economy. Henry Ford's new company, which would eventually become known as FOMOCO, (Ford Motor Company) to the residents of Detroit, or the Blue Oval, led the way and spawned General Motors and Chrysler. Growing up near Detroit, in Roseville, I lived and breathed cars as a kid. My father, Bill Hill (Wild Bill Hill to many), was a VP of sales for Dodge in the fifties and later worked for the Hurst floor-shift company. This meant I got to meet many of the famous dragster drivers and even Hurst's own Miss Golden Shifter, Linda Vaughn. A young man tends not to forget her attributes. The winters, though harsh, were often like a picture postcard, with snow-capped roofs and pine trees trimmed in white. Hudson's twelfth-floor Christmas display, a jaunt down Lakeshore Drive to see how the mansions were decorated, a Vernors' cooler on a hot summer day, the roar of the hydroplanes on the Detroit River, a lazy day spent on the Bob-Lo boat—all of this made the Motor City a grand place to live in the golden era.

We were Greasers back then in Roseville. We wore our hair in Fonzie-style waterfalls and dressed in full-length leather coats and skin-tight pants. All we wanted in life were fast cars; blond, curvy girlfriends; and jobs to keep it all going. Lucky me. I had a '57 Ford, my girl was two inches taller than I was, and I was manager of the highest volume shoe store in Detroit, Flagg Brothers, at 7 Mile and Gratiot.

I was consistently voted the most improved athlete because I was a late bloomer. Looking back, I think it was highly likely that I was allergic to wheat. This is now known as celiac disease. For me it went undiagnosed for fifty-five years. One of the characteristics is failure to thrive, or not developing on time. This was embarrassing for two reasons. First, the physical education teacher usually had the boys shower together, and around the seventh grade it became obvious if you were the only boy wearing his towel to the showers. Second, the girls were suddenly taller—much taller. It would have been obscene for me to slow dance with any of them, since, as you may recall, public breastfeeding was frowned upon in the sixties. Other characteristics of gluten intolerance are bloating, gas, diarrhea, and constant headaches. None of the aforementioned characteristics lends itself to successful dating. When my hormones finally did kick in, I threw myself into weight lifting in a nearly futile attempt to buff up and catch up for the ladies (see the gratuitous topless photo of me for proof). During a 175-pound bench press one evening, I felt a sharp pain in my chest when the bar came down. It would later prove to be one of four nonmalignant tumors removed from my chest area. This limited my future career with the International Federation of Body Builders—and I threatened my brothers and sister that I'd kill them if they told anyone I was having boob jobs. Something was wrong with me, but the doctors were unable to say anything more definitive than my hormones might be acting up.

"Fake it till you make it" has always been a way of life for me. My adolescent years were iffy for several reasons: I was four feet eleven inches in high school; I had the grade-point average that made all the others possible; and I was trying to figure out why I just couldn't digest anything. My salvation was my very cynical, warped, razor-sharp sense of humor. Simply put, I was dubbed the official class clown in 1965. I sifted everything I saw, read, and heard through the "What's funny about this?" filter. Almost everything that people believed, thought, or said made me blink quickly and think, "Really?" Years later, when I enrolled in theological school at my mother's behest, I asked one of my professors in the first week of classes, "What if the book of Genesis was really a satire, and we just didn't get it?" I envisioned Moses doing stand-up in the Catskills. Going for the joke was not a choice for me; when the talking snake entered the Garden to tempt Eve, I could hear him humming show tunes and speaking in the voice of Edward G. Robinson. This point of view proved to be very unpopular with the faculty and staff and partially led to my early departure from seminary.

However, it was during my theological studies that I learned a lesson at ten thousand feet in the air that would prove to be a game-changer later in life.

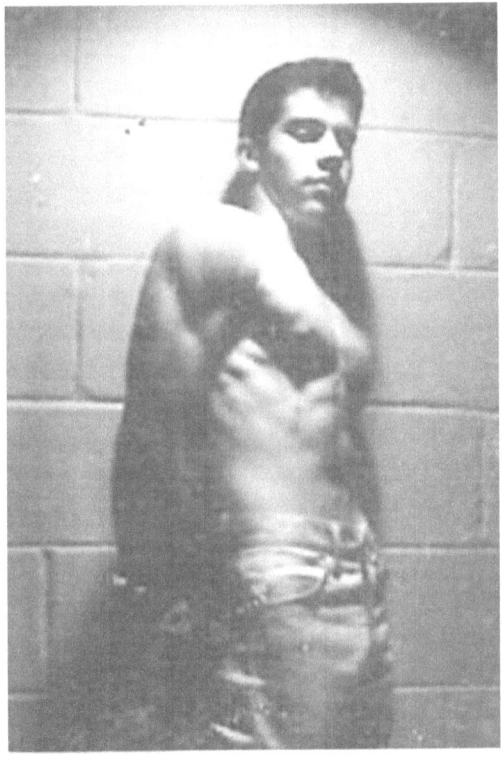

After training two years for the ladies in high school

THE KEY THAT WOULD
UNLOCK A LOT OF DOORS

When you grow up in a broken home in the 1950s, where money is scarce or mismanaged, it seems like other people's worlds are okay, but yours is not. I felt this way a lot living with my mother and three siblings. To this day, I have to fight feelings of scarcity even in the face of plenty. I recall being out with my little hoodie buddies, walking the streets late at night and looking into the windows of homes. I wasn't a Peeping Tom, looking into bedroom or bathroom windows. Instead, I was looking at families in living rooms, sitting on nice furniture and talking to one another. My family never had nice furniture, and we seldom spoke to one another unless it was with our fists. When I was growing up, my world was marked by what we weren't and what we didn't have.

My church and my mother were very interested in sending me to a Baptist college to straighten me out. Whatever did they mean? Class clowns don't need straightening out; they just need an audience. However, the unpopular war in Vietnam was brewing, and the draft was reinstated. Suddenly, I felt the call of God to enroll in theological school. Besides, this school was the only one that would take me with my grade-point average, and the church was willing to chip in for my tuition.

During my freshman year, when Thanksgiving break came I could not afford to go back to Detroit, so I planned to stay in the dorm in Owatonna, Minnesota. Al Pehl, my roommate's father, owned his own airplane and planned to fly from Rochester to Chattanooga, Tennessee, for Thanksgiving. Rusty, my roommate, asked me if I'd like to go along. I had never been on an airplane. Heck, yeah!

Fortunately for me, it was a Beechcraft Bonanza, a four-seater, a real beauty. I was fascinated with the preflight checks, communications with the tower, and takeoff. What a rush! The power and noise were so intense. Once we leveled off at about ten thousand feet, Al Pehl asked, "You boys mind if I play a cassette tape while we fly?" Like we had a choice? It wasn't like we could go for a walk instead. "No," we said in unison. Rusty and I looked at each other, thinking "Oh, boy, here we go, probably a sermon."

For the next couple of hours, I listened in rapt attention to Earl Nightingale's *Lead the Field* series. I would never be the same. He spoke of worlds I had never seen. No one in my world, not my parents, my teachers, my high-school counselors, my pastor, or my theology professors, had ever spoken of having the freedom and personal power to avoid poverty and dependency. Earl said that during the Great Depression, most men would do anything for work. Then he gave several examples of people who not only survived but also prospered in the worst of times. He talked about becoming "the man on the white horse." So far, I had been the boy on the black mutt. I asked Rusty's dad if I could borrow the tapes after we returned, and he lent me the tape player and the twelve tapes. I devoured them, listening night and day until I nearly had the entire series memorized. I had no earthly idea what I was going to do with that information. But six years later, these lessons made all the difference in my life.

My propensity to see life as if I were stuck in a *Saturday Night Live* sketch got me through college and seminary with some sanity left. Years later, when I was diagnosed with stage-three embroyonal cell carcinoma, I have to say that there were aspects of my cancer experience that were hysterical to me, and I believe my sense of comedy was a factor in my recovery. It is my belief that if one can remain entertained and optimistic, one's recovery may be more likely. Disease may have a harder time succeeding in a body that has a humorous mindset, even if the body isn't a paragon of resistance and strength. So let me tell you my story, in all its gory detail, with the hope that it may inspire you to wellness and laughter. Hang on to your butts . . .

After I graduated from Bible college with a BA in theology and English, I was working full time as an administrator at the New Ulm Christian School in New Ulm, Minnesota. During that time, I went to several doctors to find out why I was getting more of the chest tumors I had gotten in high school. One doctor said, "Well, since it seems to be confined to the breast area, I suggest we do a double mastectomy—you know, just remove all the breast tissue and muscle. You'll have a 'V' on your chest, like a 'V' for 'victory,' heh, heh." He said this with a straight face, and he charged me for the visit. How much should that advice cost? Why do some doctors wonder why people tend to not trust them and are a tad litigious?

Early one September morning in 1974, I was scratching where men tend to scratch at that time of day when I felt pain. Searing pain, the kind of pain that would end my horseback-riding career indefinitely. It's one thing to have your chest hurt, quite another to have the family jewels yodeling in agony. We've all heard stories about wartime torture where POWs vow never to tell anything until their captors move below the belt—and then they sing like the fat lady at the opera. It's primordial. We are programmed to protect future generations at all costs. I went to several more doctors until one said, "We may be dealing with something more than nonmalignant tumors. I'm going to refer you to the Mayo Clinic. It's only about a three-hour drive, okay?" Suddenly I was no longer worried about a "V" on my chest for "victory." I was starting to worry about an "E" for "eunuch."

OCD HEAVEN: THE MAYO CLINIC

For those of you who've been diagnosed at one time or another with obsessive-compulsive disorder (OCD), you would kill for a chance to go to the Mayo Clinic. It is, quite simply, OCD nirvana. It is the cleanest, most organized facility on Earth. It's sterile, it's white, everything's at right angles, and there's a "just-showered" atmosphere. It's like having a day off for an OCD person, because almost nothing needs fixing. It's an assembly line like Henry Ford built, only neater. It's color-coded, easily marked, and clear as a bell.

After being tested, poked, prodded, and x-rayed for three days, I was ushered into Dr. Alfred Bertagnol's office, which was unlike any other doctor's office I had ever visited. There were no tongue depressors, ear flashlights, anatomy charts, or yellowed degrees for wall groupings. This office was purely modern and expensively decorated. I liked this doctor for some reason. He didn't talk with the editorial "we," look over the top of his glasses and grunt at me, or say dumb things that neither of us really believed. He was nondescript in appearance, not tall, not short, not handsome, and not homely. Like me.

"Mr. Hill," he began, "you have had a lot of tests this week. Unfortunately, the biopsy we took was positive. The tumor is malignant."

"Uh, say what?" I said incredulously. "Doc, come on. I'm twenty-three years old. Can these tests give false positives?"

"Not likely," he said, glancing down at about twenty-five pages. "We took several samples, and they were all positive. You are, of course, free to seek a second medical opinion, but I'd stake my diploma on this one. Your cancer is high-grade embryonal cell carcinoma, and now we need to know if it has spread and, if so, how far. Day after tomorrow, I've scheduled you for some major exploratory surgery. I'll remove all the lymph nodes down one side near your spine. If none of them are malignant, I'll stop there. If some are, then I'll need to remove the other side as well and any other cancerous areas we may find. It is a very serious operation and very lengthy. This is standard procedure in cases like this. Any questions?"

Was he kidding? Any questions? How about, oh, I don't know, "Why me?" or, "Who said I wanted to have this surgery? What do you mean, you've 'scheduled' me? Can't we negotiate this thing? I'm the principal of a parochial school, for crying out loud. I work for God!"

The next couple of days were equally miserable. I had a liquid diet, an enema, shots, pills, and *that* shave. Too soon for me, the boys in white flopped my drugged carcass onto the gurney, and off we went down the hall, to the right, through the swinging doors, and into what looked like a tiled ballpark. It had packed bleachers and was lighted to the max. The anesthesiologist told me what he was doing as he went. When the second needle hit my shoulder, I was determined to follow his instructions and count to ten.

One . . . two . . . three . . . four . . . five . . .

Six hours of surgery cause enormous trauma to the body. Imagine doctors making an opening in your abdomen almost sixteen inches long. In order to get to your spine, they have to move your stomach, intestines, and who knows what else out of the way. Did they take snapshots to remember how everything is supposed to look when they're done? Car mechanics do.

After that kind of surgery, the human body does not want to restart very quickly. If you add up all the time I was chemically unconscious, it might have been as much as eight or nine hours. Of course, I was on so much morphine after the surgery that it had to be three full days before I felt I had rejoined the land of the living.

To add insult to injury, they started working my lungs right away with what they called blow bottles. The object of the game is to move colored water from one bottle to the other by blowing on a curling tube. Sounds easy enough, but when your entire gut has been filleted like a giant musky on the shore of Lake Michigan, it's a bit tough. Each breath I drew caused intense pain. Like a drug addict living on the street or under a bridge, I needed a fix for pain, and I needed it fast! About every five hours, the nurse would come with her *Magical Mystery Tour* needle and send me uptown. Then, within an hour, the pain would begin to creep back in, like a thief waiting in the shadows, closing in slowly. By the fifth hour, my abdomen was on fire, and I was prepared to sell my body to science for a single shot of morphine. I wish I could tell you that I just thought positive thoughts and the pain went away. Every blow-dried motivational speaker insists that the key to life is focus and that what the mind can conceive and believe . . . Yeah, well, I was focused, all right, on a needle.

After a day or two, once I got the blow bottles moving, the nurses hauled my crumpled butt out of bed and said I needed to walk to prevent pneumonia. Ever try to walk when you have a sixteen-inch incision and you're connected to a Hemovac, IVs, and a catheter? One of the pictures included is of me trying to push the "needle cart" down the hall. It was a bit like jogging without skin on the bottoms of your feet.

After a few days, it was time to huddle again with the doc.

"We need to do a test called a lymphangiogram," he said, as though I'd know what that was, "to determine if it has metastasized or spread. Another doctor will perform this test, but I'll get a full report. How are you feeling?"

"Doing what you do, Doc," I panned. "Keeping everyone in stitches."

The exam room was like all the rest: clean, sterile, and indifferent. As I lay there, a metal plate was inserted into the top of my foot—without Novocain, since it would interfere with the dye. They proceeded to inject dye slowly with needles. Did I mention this was without Novocain?

These little metal plates were inserted just under the skin, and dye was pumped into my lymph system so that it would rise up my leg. A large television monitor showed the path of the dye. The first few attempts to insert the plates failed, and I have multiple scars on the tops of both feet to prove it. Finally they succeeded, and, sure enough, the screen showed the dye beginning to rise. The technicians high-fived one another as though a guy weren't lying on the table with blood dripping from his toes.

After the results of this lymphangiogram came in, Dr. Bertagnol scheduled a consultation. Something was up, and it wasn't my morale.

This was a bit like sneaking a peek at your bank balance after the stock market has crashed. You have a feeling of what the truth might be; you just don't want to see it or hear about it.

"Well," he said, lounging on the edge of my bed, "we found positive nodes in your neck and in your feet—so your cancer is clearly systemic at this point."

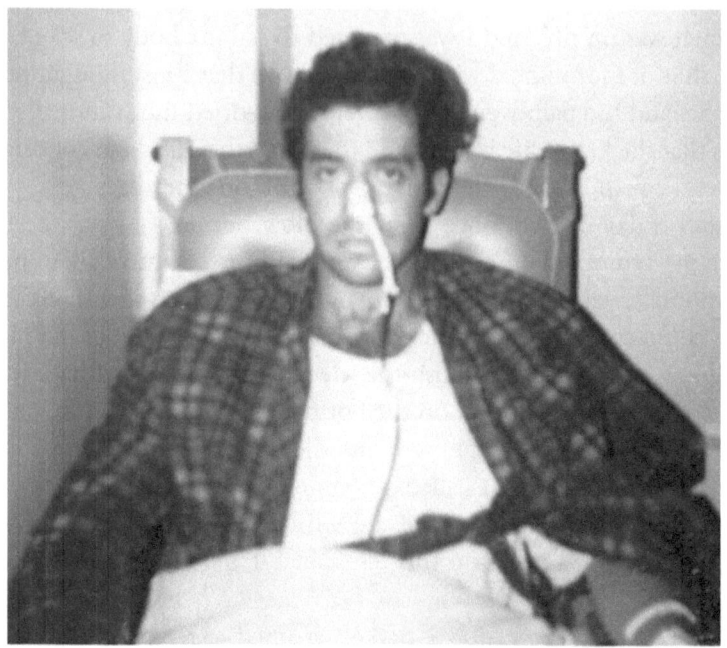

A few days after surgery, trying to sit up

He glanced at the stomach pump taped to the bridge of my nose and pushed it around a little. Then he excused himself and left the room as though he hadn't just told me that I was steeped from head to toe in cancer. After a minute or so, he came back with a nurse, who was carrying a larger hose. This could not be good news. The circumference of any object about to be inserted up your nose is of primary importance. Bigger is not better.

"This," he shouted, pointing at my nose as he scolded her (or the staff in general, who could hear down the hall), "is clearly too small. Whoever inserted this after surgery was not paying attention. Kindly remove this thing and insert that one," he said, pointing to the hose in her hand.

He quickly turned on his heel, saying he would see me tomorrow morning, and stomped out of the room. I never did get to react to the "systemic spread" comment. The nurse leaned over me and removed the tape from the bridge of my nose. "They put this in when you were under sedation so you felt nothing," she said. "It's quite uncomfortable to remove it and insert one while you're conscious. I'll be as careful and as gentle as I can, okay?"

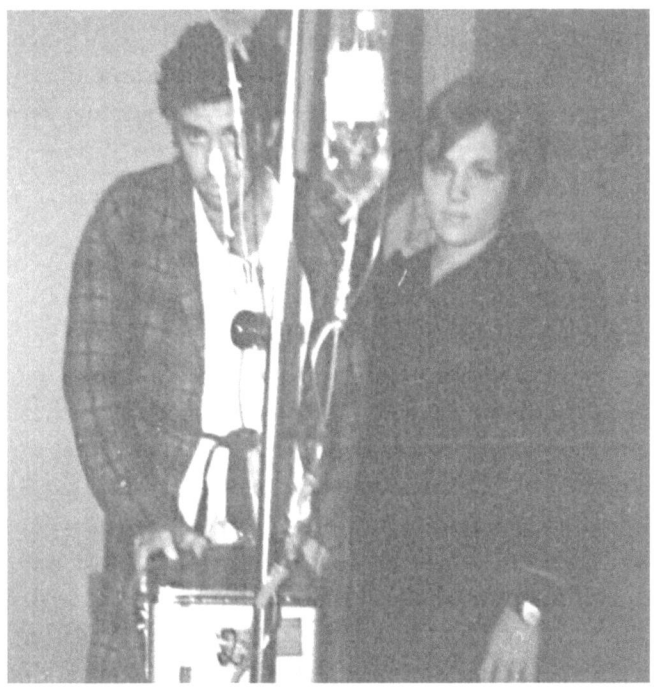

Trying to walk to avoid pneumonia

What followed felt like she was pulling my toes up through my stomach and out my nose. I began gagging and coughing, which put a strain on hundreds of stitches. Tears poured from my eyes. In seconds it was out, and I glared at her like she'd done it for spite.

"You did well," she said. "Putting this larger one in is more challenging. I'm going to insert this tube through your nose. When you feel it hit the back of your throat, you'll have the urge to gag. As much as you can, start swallowing, okay, Sweetie?"

"Sure, Lover-Lump."

She leaned over me, and I can assure you that at this point in time I was not trying to sneak a peek at her cleavage. I felt the tube enter my nose. In seconds, it was scratching the back of my throat. When I started to gag and retch, she began shouting in my ear, "Swallow, swallow, swallow!"

When she kept pushing this hose (the size of a Detroit sewer pipe) down my throat, I reached up and grabbed her by the front of her clinical smock and screeched, "Are you trying to kill me before the cancer does?"

My wife ran from the room in tears while Nurse Mildred Ratched finished taping things down. She gave me a liberal dose of liquid La La Land, but before I drifted off to sleep I remember thinking, *Trying to help me at this point is like rearranging the deck chairs on the Titanic. It keeps you busy, but it isn't doing much.*

Speaking of not accomplishing anything, let's fast-forward about thirty-five years, when I discovered the seeming futility of what had been done for me at Mayo. This, you're going to love.

About twelve of us were sliding around on Chicago's icy roads near O'Hare after the Delta jet failed to leave the gate due to "mechanical difficulties." This usually meant there weren't enough people on board to make the flight pay. We were issued a generous voucher for a six-dollar sandwich and a midnight ride to a crummy hotel, where we'd spend the night until a six o'clock flight the next morning. There we were, sledding our way to the hotel, when one of the passengers decided to be the activities coordinator for Chez Minivan. "Okay," she chirped, "let's go around the bus and tell what we do for a living and where we're headed. I'll start. My name is Shirley, and . . ."

We sat through twenty minutes of tortured testimonials until it came time for the guy next to me to speak. "I'm Dr. Barker," he said, clearing his throat. "I'm a urologist specializing in cancer surgery, oncology . . ." Suddenly, a voice from the back of the bus yelled, "Cancer? How's business, Doc? Everyone's got it these days!" The doctor paused, turned around, and answered, "Business is booming! I'm so busy I only take the more dramatic cases now."

The hair stood up on the back of my neck. I couldn't help myself, and it wasn't a punchline I wanted to deliver. "Maybe you operated on me then, Doc," I said, "and helped your business boom and all. I had radical abdominal surgery for stage-three high-grade embryonal cell carcinoma. It was pretty sensational back in the seventies; they even posted flyers in the hallway at Mayo for younger doctors to watch from the viewing deck."

"Yeah," he said, yawning. "We don't even do that procedure anymore. It didn't accomplish much, and it had complications."

Didn't accomplish much? Six hours of surgery and hundreds of thousands of dollars?

SELLING THE FAMILY

Some challenges in life are insurmountable, and no amount of "glass is half full" mental gymnastics or rhetoric quite helps. When my family members learned the extent of the cancer, most of them flew into Rochester for a family meeting. We met at my in-laws' home in Stewartville, Minnesota. There was a late October chill in the air, a nice fire was crackling in the fireplace, and the smell of freshly popped popcorn filled the house; this was straight out of a Norman Rockwell painting. What I heard the loudest was what wasn't being said. How do you talk to someone who's dying? I was afraid I'd get questions like these:

"So," my brother said casually, "have you given any thought to that gold watch Pop gave you?"

"Bro, have you ever wondered if you can actually feel the surgery even though they knock you out?"

"Can I borrow some cash? I mean, it's not like you'll need the money back or anything. Just sayin'."

It was a very tense evening, though it was pretty typical of my family to say nothing about the obvious. I was down to 125 pounds and crumpled up on a Barcalounger like an old man. They all said I looked great and that they were sure everything was going to be A-OK. Geez . . .

The following day, we met with a chemotherapist, who suggested ten treatments of actinomycin D. I asked him if he had any patient referrals or testimonials I could talk to or read. You know, a little due diligence.

Nada.

I told him I wanted a day to sleep on it, to which he said, "You don't have the luxury of time. If you have any chance at all of a recovery, we have to start this now."

That night, Doug McLachlan, the pastor from the Christian school where I worked, drove up and handed me some mail. One letter in particular caught my attention, because it was from a Pastor John Ballentine. John was a fundamentalist Baptist who was knee-deep in John Bircher meetings and conspiracy theories. His letter basically told me to run, not walk, out of the Mayo Clinic and go somewhere where they understood the human body and nutrition. His "somewhere" turned out to be Tijuana, Mexico, where a Dr. Ernesto Contreras was getting a lot of press for giving stage-three and -four cancer patients a substance called Laetrile, or vitamin B17. Today it is generally referred to as amygdalin, which is still illegal in the States. He claimed that this substance, along with some catalytic enzymes and a special diet, was making terminal patients better.

DECISIONS, DECISIONS . . .

Do I believe THE MAYO CLINIC or a baptist pastor that had a tendency to see conspiracies under every bush? How do we make difficult decisions? Don't you often wish you were smarter? I sure do.

I remember I was at work one day when a fellow worker came in looking absolutely ill. She was walking as though in great pain. I asked her what was wrong? She sighed, pursed her lips and said, "I just had some lung x-rays taken because I've had a persistent cough. The doctor thinks he's found a spot on my lung—and it could be cancer."

For the next couple of days she would tear-up at the slightest discussion and at one point she just left work and went home to go to bed. She was waiting for all of her tests to come in before she was scheduled to go in for consultation.

The next afternoon she came bounding into work smiling and giving everyone hugs. Her story was that the doctor had read the wrong x-rays but now gave her a clean bill of health. After letting everyone know how happy she was, she announced that she was going to find the nearest bar, order a very large cocktail or two and have a cigarette. My question was, what was going on in her brain that made her so sick when she was apparently given bad information by the doctor?

Are we programmed to believe bad news more than we believe good news? In his book, *Abundance*, by Peter H. Diamandis (MD and Ph. D), he says, "Since nothing is more critical to the brain than survival, the first filter most of this incoming information is filtered through is the amygdala. The amygdala is an almond-shaped sliver of the temporal lobe responsible for primal emotions like rage, hate and fear. It's our early warning system, an organ always on high alert whose job is to find anything in our environment that could threaten survival . . . what all of this means is that once the amygdala begins hunting bad news, it's mostly going to find bad news."

This may be why bad news travels so fast and why it's hard to believe there might be hope. All of our family, friends, and even the doctors have one of these amygdalas and are prone to deliver bad news whenever possible. They and we can't help it. This "fight or flight" mechanism may have kept us from being eaten by saber-toothed tigers, but it doesn't help us much in modern times when we try to separate real from imagined dangers.

Secondly, there is the tendency to believe anyone we perceive is an authority. When an authority figure says we have a terminal illness we are not likely to stop believing that because a friend tells us it isn't so.

How in the world was I going to make a decision based on the input I had?

But then I got to thinking. It was fairly clear to me that I wasn't going to be buying any green bananas anyway and that my chemotherapist had been colder than a mother-in-law's kiss. After reading all the literature in the envelope, I decided to get the family together and get their opinion—you know, a family meeting.

Bahahahahahahah.

"Ricky," my brother Sam (Sam Hill, honest) shouted, "You're an idiot! You've always been an idiot, and this only proves it. No one in their right mind would even consider leaving Mayo and going to *Tijuana*. Are you crazy? Do they give you a tequila worm as part of the diet?"

"Don't hold back, Sam," I said. "Just tell me straight what you really think."

I looked over at my dad, who had flown in from Tyler, Texas. He just nodded and said, "Ditto."

By now the ladies were in tears, the pastor was busy looking at his shoes, and Norman Rockwell grabbed his canvas and headed for the door.

"Okay," I said. "I'm sensing a slightly negative vibe here. But it's *my* life, after all. If I make a mistake, it can cost me everything." I looked around. "And 'oops' won't quite cover it."

Only the pastor and my father-in-law thought it was a good idea for me to leave Mayo and go to Tijuana. The next morning, I went into the clinic and met again with the chemotherapist. I told him that I was considering going to the Oasis of Hope Hospital in Tijuana. He got a wry grin on his face and said, "Well, it *is* warm in Tijuana this time of year . . ."

The next logical step was to call the clinic in Mexico and talk with one of the doctors. Dr. Contreras was the founder and the one getting all the press (even an article in *People* magazine). When I finally got through to the clinic, his niece, who was a receptionist at the time, answered my call. I explained my case to her, and she apparently sensed my urgency.

I asked, "Can Dr. Contreras be reached by phone?"

"No, he's at a friend's house for dinner tonight."

"Well, I respect his privacy," I argued, "but I'm twenty-three years old, and I haven't had any chemotherapy or radiation. My cancer is stage three already and spreading fast. Could I speak with him for just five minutes tonight?"

"Well," she began, "your case sounds good. Okay, give me your number, and I'll call him. But please, don't talk with him more than five minutes, okay?"

"Agreed," I said quickly.

Our phone rang about fifteen minutes later, and I picked up. The now-famous physician said, "Hello, Richard. This is Dr. Contreras."

"Dr. Contreras, I'm sorry to bother you on your personal time."

"That's okay. What can I do for you?" he said in a surprisingly unruffled tone. I relaxed a little.

"I have stage-three embryonal cell carcinoma. I've had nearly ten hours of surgeries at the Mayo Clinic but no chemotherapy or radiation. I feel pretty well except for all that surgery. Is it worth it to try Laetrile?"

"Well, I haven't seen your records, but we have treated others like you with good success. Can you travel?"

"Yes."

"Could you be an outpatient, or would you require hospitalization?"

"I'm at home now, so I don't think I need to be in the hospital."

"When can you come, and can you bring your records with you?"

"In a couple of days, and I'll get my records."

"Okay, Richard. Tomorrow I'll make an appointment to see you Thursday morning. You get checked in Wednesday, and they'll run some tests on you. After we review your records and the tests we run, we'll decide if Laetrile is an option."

"Okay," I said. "I'll see you Thursday, then. Thank you for calling me back."

How were we going to pay for all this? Pastor McLachlan drove back to New Ulm that night, and the people of the First Baptist Church raised (or borrowed) all the money I needed to make the trip with my father-in-law. You have to understand the sacrifice these good people made. The First Baptist Church was, at that time, a small congregation of fewer than two hundred people. Most were either farmers or blue-collar workers in the local Kraft Foods factory. They raised what would be by today's standards about $50,000 to send me to Oasis. Hardly a day goes by that I don't think about what they did for me. If someday I wind up rich, perhaps I can return the favor by sending someone like me to Oasis—you know, paying it forward.

What can you do if you don't have the cash available? The Oasis of Hope hospital has a couple of programs to assist those who need to borrow money for treatment, and there is a very limited amount of money available through donations to http://www.canceraidresearch.org. For this reason, I'm donating 50 percent of my net income from the sale of this book to help some people who simply have no money for treatment. The money will go only to patients without resources, and this will be determined by Oasis. Here's another idea: if you have a large church or temple, I will waive my speaking fee (except expenses) to speak at a service in order to help you raise money for one of your members with cancer.

With the money in hand, two days later my father-in-law and I were on a plane to San Diego, headed straight down the rabbit hole.

PART TWO

Tijuana, Mexico 1974

THE RABBIT HOLE

My father-in-law, Les, was a very resourceful man. He owned a heavy-equipment company that built roads and dams. He took over a month off work to travel with me, enabling me to take the trip. When we got to San Diego, we didn't have a place to stay, so we checked into a cheap hotel near the border in San Ysidro. At least the sheets were clean, and it had a phone. Les called Tim LaHaye's mega church and asked if there might be someone from the church with whom we could stay. Later that evening, our room phone rang, and an elderly woman began speaking so loudly that I had to hold the phone away from my ear to save my eardrum.

"My name is Soldier Burfurd," she announced, "and I'd be delighted to pick you up tomorrow morning at seven o'clock sharp. Pack your bags, because I have a place for you two to stay—nothing fancy, but there are hot showers, and I'll take care of the rest." The next morning, I'd discover that Soldier was about five feet six inches tall and all of 105 pounds soaking wet. She wore her hair in a severe bun and sported horn-rimmed glasses from the sixties. Her lipstick was smeared a little above her lip and always seemed to be on her front teeth. She had been married forever to a now-deceased retired navy admiral. After she found out Les was in the navy in World War II, they got along just fine. When she barked an order at us, he replied in an ear-splitting fashion, "Ma'am, yes, ma'am!" You think that's strange? Keep reading.

She picked us up at 0700 hours on the button. We were waiting in the lobby, and she pulled up in her beige, slightly dented Dodge Dart. After crisply shaking our hands, she personally loaded our bags into the trunk, and off we went. My best guess was that she was crowding eighty years old. Just a guess.

We spent the day getting settled, which meant going with Soldier to a local health-food store. Not only did I weigh less than 125 pounds by then, but also I was walking hunched over like an old man. The abdominal pain kept me from standing up straight or sitting for any length of time. When I was in a car, I tried to lie down on the backseat. Soldier shouted at me in the backseat, driving with one eye on the road and one eye on me in the rearview mirror.

"Your world is about to change, young man," she barked at me. Then she turned to Les. "You've got to make sure he only eats what's on the diet sheet they'll give him, and no cheating! Is that understood?"

"Ma'am, yes, ma'am!" Les barked back.

"Good," she continued. "Because if I find out you've been cheating on the diet, I'll no longer help you."

She pulled into the parking lot of a 1974 health-food store. I was used to Kroger stores, which had nice, wide aisles and fruit polished and stacked attractively. This place was a dump. There were shoppers who looked like they hadn't eaten or slept in months, wearing wrinkled granny dresses and gross flip-flops revealing blackened chipped toenails. To make matters worse, they were leaning over open barrels with small shovels, loading food into paper bags. Soldier grabbed a couple of baskets, one for Les and one for herself. I hobbled along behind them trying to keep pace.

"Rule number one," she said, loudly enough for the store across the street to hear, "no chemicals. Everything Rick eats needs to be as natural as possible. If it had a face, don't eat it." With that diatribe out of the way, she proceeded to load things into the baskets that I wouldn't even step in—much less eat. I had never seen or eaten an avocado before, but that was about to change. Her idea of a sandwich was sliced avocado on organic bread with tomatoes and sprouts. Today, I love that sandwich. Back then? Not so much.

Why was it that health-food stores, especially in the seventies, looked like refugee camps? There were rail-thin people walking around humming Ravi Shankar tunes, and I'm pretty sure we three were the only ones in the store wearing any underwear. The other shoppers said things like "Totally" and "Oh, wow, man." I felt like Michael J. Fox's young Republican character from *Family Ties* at a DNC. We passed a rack displaying enema bags, and Soldier said, "You'll find out about these soon enough." We returned home that night to a tiny two-bedroom apartment that Soldier had borrowed from some people who were out of the country for a while.

"This will do," she announced as we walked into the dark living room. "There are two bedrooms but only one bathroom. Let's get these groceries put away, and I'll make you boys something to eat."

"Something to eat" turned out to be one of her avocado whiz-pop-bang dealie-bobs, organic lentil soup, and carrot juice. Everything seemed tasteless to me, because none of it was fried or salted.

My mother, Freddie (not kidding again), was born on Sand Mountain, Alabama. We grew up on soul food. There wasn't a food she couldn't improve if she could get it bubbling in lard. She could fry Jell-O and make it taste better. When she got home from work, she'd slice off a slab of lard from the brick that sat on the back of the stove. She'd drop it into a large black iron skillet and decide what to fry for dinner. At least once a week, we had white gravy on white bread, fried potatoes, and bacon for dinner. On Sundays, we got pork chops or a pot roast, cornbread, and a big pot of Kentucky Wonder beans. This southern food was delicious, because most of it was fried, heavily salted, and cooked to death. Yum!

When Soldier turned her back, I donated part of my carrot juice to a potted plant and slid my sandwich on Les's plate. He could and would eat anything put in front of him. Having been born and raised in Minnesota, he'd eaten things like lutefisk and huge chunks of blue cheese. Avocado was a walk in the park for him. If only it didn't look so much like diaper poop . . .

After Soldier cleared the table and washed the dishes, she turned and said, "I'll pick you up at six o'clock sharp tomorrow morning." Then she headed for the door. "Don't be late. We have to get to the clinic early to get a low number."

"A low number?" I asked.

"You'll see soon enough." With that, she let the door slam behind her. Everything in Soldier's world was on a need-to-know basis. I didn't sleep well that night. I figured it was my last night on Earth, with any luck.

LIFE AMONG THE DYING

The little Dodge Dart bounced along in the passing lane on the 805 south, going fifteen miles under the speed limit. I was in too much pain to care, and Les wasn't about to tangle with Soldier. Soon we arrived at the border. When we pulled up to the little border-patrol booth, Soldier gave the guard the evil eye, as if to say, "Try me." He waved us through without a question.

I'll never forget that first trip from the border down to the clinic. The poverty visible from the main drag as you head toward the ocean is heart wrenching. How can a country be so close to San Diego and look like this? We drove in silence, looking at row after row of tin buildings and the graffiti covering every stucco wall. But the closer we got to the hospital, the better the view and neighborhood got. Finally we got our first glimpse of what was at that time called the Good Samaritan Clinic. Nestled right across the street from the bullring in a small group of commercial buildings, only a block from the ocean, the clinic consisted of a main building and several small, connected huts. Once we went through the doors, nothing was the least bit familiar.

We walked into the main area and saw a reception desk on the far side of the room. There were almost fifty people milling around, waiting to be seen.

"You find a place to sit or lie down, Rick," Les said, "and I'll get us checked in." I found a couple of chairs I could push together in order to lie down. When this proved to be too uncomfortable, I sat up and saw a large throw rug under a painting of The Good Samaritan and like the family dog, curled up on the rug and tried to sleep. As long as we got there early, I could claim that spot and wait my turn. At least a hundred people passed through that waiting room throughout the day, trying to be seen. I've never in my life seen so many desperate people in one place, except for the night I saw the Flying Wallendas fall at the Shrine Circus in Detroit. This clinic seemed like a hospital in a war zone. I saw people with half-missing faces and missing limbs, and there were lots of women with completely flat chests. After several hours, a nurse came to me and said with a heavy Spanish accent, "Please follow me for some tests."

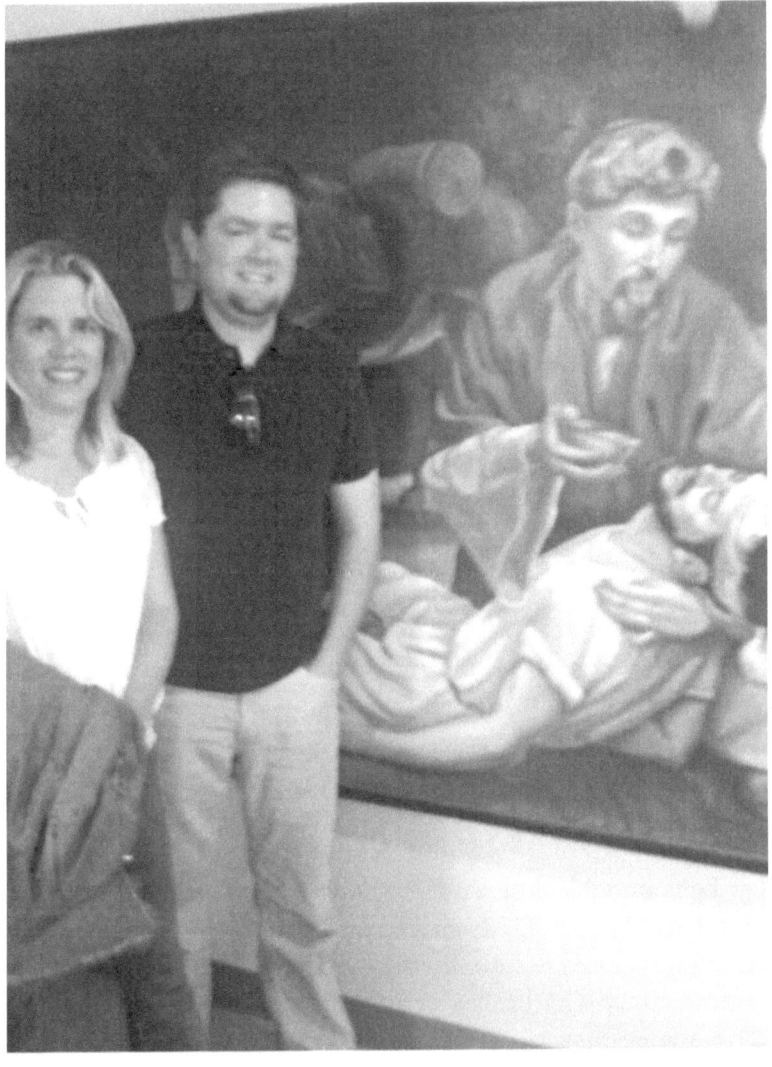

My kids, Heather and Rick standing in front of the very same painting of the Good Samaritan now hanging in the cafeteria instead of the lobby.

Les and I were emerging from an exam room when we saw a tall Mexican man walking toward us. I had seen pictures of Dr. Contreras, and this had to be him. As he approached, I said, "Dr. Contreras, it's Rick Hill and Les Bardwell from Minnesota. We talked two days ago?"

You never forget the first time he smiles at you. It's a smile of connection, with no pretense. He shook my hand and Les's hand firmly, with both of his. He wore a white lab coat with his name printed on the pocket. Like so many Mexican gentlemen, he'd combed his hair straight back and had a well-trimmed mustache.

Dr. Contreras received postgraduate training at the Children's Hospital in Boston. He served as the chief pathologist at the Army Hospital Mexico City and was professor of histology and pathology at the Mexican Army Medical School.

"Have you had your blood work done yet?" he asked. We nodded. "If so, follow me to my office. I have to leave early tomorrow for Italy to deliver some papers on our work to their medical society. I'm so glad I ran into you, because I will be gone for at least two weeks. Dr. Lopez will be your doctor. You're in good hands with him. He and I will speak every single night, so if there are problems or questions about your case, I'll hear about them that very day. You and I will visit again when I get back."

We sat and chatted about my case, and he promised he would review my records before he left the next day.

We went back to the waiting room for a couple more hours until my turn came for treatment. The treatment back then was simply a three-gram injection of Laetrile and a retention enema of Wobe Mugos catalytic enzymes. I got used to hearing, "Roll on your side . . . Relax . . . Okay, don't release this for at least twenty minutes or as long as you can wait."

Every morning we arrived around seven o'clock. If necessary, we'd wait for a good part of the day to see a doctor and get the treatment. Each Friday, I got a double dose, or a six-gram injection, and did not come in on Saturday or Sunday. Dr. Contreras preached the gospel at the clinic for all those who wanted to hear. Les and I did not attend any services there but instead visited Tim LaHaye's church in San Diego.

Over the next few weeks, I underwent periodic tests, lung x-rays, and nutritional counseling at the clinic. Around the fifth day, a nurse took me into a room and said, "It's time to start your detoxification in order to rid your body of these poisons as much as we can."

"How do we do that?" I asked.

"Have you ever changed the water in the radiator of your car?" she asked.

"Sure."

"How did you do it?"

"Well," I said, trying to look mechanical, "I took off the radiator cap, unscrewed the butterfly cap at the bottom, shoved a garden hose in the top, and turned on the water."

"Exactly!" she exclaimed. "That's kind of what we're going to do!" I looked at her, blinked a few hundred times, then asked, "So where does the hose go?"

Soldier had been right at the health-food store when she said I'd find out soon enough what enema bags were for. That day, I had my first high colonic, followed by several coffee enemas—no cream or sugar. For those of you who don't know what a high colonic is all about, imagine yourself waterskiing very fast and then just sitting down . . .

There is no way to describe what life in the clinic's lobby was like for those three weeks. I called it Lobby Lore. We'd all left families and friends behind and entered a strange new country, and we were together to fight for a common cause. Like men at war, if we lost our battle, we would lose everything. There was nothing we wouldn't tell one another. For many of us, these would be the last friends we'd ever make. We were pretty aware of it when someone didn't return or was sent home to die.

One day, a family of Amish farmers entered the lobby like rush-hour cars moving in a single-file line. The large bearded father came in first, carrying what looked like a fifteen-year-old boy in his arms. His son's legs were swollen to four or five times their normal size. Behind him came his mother and two sisters with their white lace caps and long dresses. The man laid his son down on some chairs that patients had vacated. Dr. Lopez came out into the lobby, examined the boy, and spoke to the farmer in hushed tones. Dr. Lopez began shaking his head and placed his hand on the man's shoulder before walking away. The father picked up his son with weathered hands and slowly walked to the doors. The boy's mother and sisters were openly crying as they followed him. They had traveled thousands of miles to do all they could for someone they loved; but it was too late. There was not a dry eye in the lobby. My guess is that they had called ahead, heard from the doctors that it was too late, but decided to come anyway.

Every day there were unforgettable sights, sounds, and odors. One day, I began talking to a woman who was about forty years old. Meeting a new person there was like meeting an inmate in prison; we asked one another some version of "What'er ya in for?" We talked for a few minutes, and then she said, "See?" She pulled her shirt up to her neck and exposed bare flesh that was a mass of deep scars and angry red skin. I nearly passed out. Whoever did that surgery should be shot. My scar was long and red, but it sure didn't look like that.

One night, one of my stitches began to itch, and then it got infected. What were we going to do? It was late, and Les and I were alone in an unfamiliar apartment. We found some rubbing alcohol and tweezers. Les lanced the site with the edge of the tweezers, found the infected stitch, pulled it out, and cut if off with a razor blade. Surgery. We coated the site in alcohol and slapped a Band-Aid on it.

No problem. Yankee ingenuity in action.

THE MYSTERY
OF THE SANTA ANA WIND

During the second week, we headed to Denny's for dinner. The car radio said a Santa Ana wind was blowing in and dropping the humidity like a rock. I didn't feel well at all. We asked to see the cook and requested that he prepare some steamed vegetables and a baked potato. We would rather have eaten at Anthony's Fish Grotto, but money was short. Denny's would have to do. Soldier didn't know we were eating at Denny's, because Les had borrowed a car in that first week from an old navy buddy of his named Curtis, who lived in San Clemente. I'll never forget when Soldier drove us up there to get the car. Curtis looked at me and said, "So that's what cancer looks like, huh? Well, if I ever get it, I'm just going to keep eating so I never look like that." I guess you can be a good navy seaman without being overly sensitive. But now that we had this car, Soldier was off duty, and we could slack off a bit. We saw her a few more times while I was there, and, of course, she was there to see us off when we left. Love is spelled S-O-L-D-I-E-R, huh?

After I had a few bites of dinner that night, my head began to swim; and when I looked up, the room began to dim. I said to Les, "I'm losing it—not sure what's wrong, but I'm going down . . ."

Les must have jumped up and caught me, because the next thing I remember, he was carrying me out of Denny's toward the car. When we got to the house, he put me on the bed, knelt down beside me, and began praying for me out loud. I closed my eyes and fell fast asleep.

I dreamed Les and I were walking in the neighborhood where we were staying. While we walked, I saw some trash piled at the end of a driveway. Sitting on top of a trash container was a light-blue portable humidifier—the kind you fill with water and plug in. When I woke from my nap, I got up and found Les reading in the living room.

"Man, that was weird," I said. "What happened at Denny's?" After he relayed the story, I asked if we could go for a short walk. We left the apartment and walked around the block. When we got to the backside of the block, some trash was piled at the end of a driveway—and sitting on top of the trash barrel was that same blue humidifier. I told Les what I had dreamed, and he said, "Well, I think the dry wind was too much for you, and you need humidity. God put this here for us to use. Obviously no one wants it, sitting out here in the trash like this."

"You think it actually works?" I asked.

We took it home, filled it with water, and put it in my bedroom. It worked like new.

You tell me. What happened? I've never had anything like that happen to me before or since, but I can't deny that it happened. Coincidence? A miracle? In true Rick Hill fashion, when we were walking away from the trash pile, I could hear the theme song from *The Twilight Zone* in my head and Rod Serling saying, "Imagine a young man caught in a struggle for his life who suddenly wakes up and finds himself in *the twilight zone*." Music up, and fade to commercial.

THE PINK ELEPHANT
IN THE ROOM

Sometimes the obvious never gets discussed. One reason everyone who goes to Oasis doesn't get well is that few show up until their cancer is already classified as stage four. Their bodies have been damaged beyond repair. Other times, people like me show up who is not yet stage four or who have not had a lot of chemo and radiation. But after a while, I noticed that several of the patients in the lobby would walk across the street for a smoke. And though we were given a very strict diet sheet to follow, often I'd see patients go to some of the local eateries near the beach and order food that was clearly not part of our diet. I wondered why anyone would go all the way to Tijuana, spend all that money, and then not follow the program? Didn't they want to live? Then I got to thinking about myself. Why was *I* there? One doctor at the clinic believed that we are all born with cancer cells and that circumstances like stress, a toxic diet, or a tragic event depress the immune system and allows the cancer cells to multiply. If these people wouldn't even stop smoking or stay on a diet to get well, I had to ask myself if they thought their lives were worth saving.

Which leads me to ask you the question I had to ask myself so long ago: "Is *your* life worth saving?"

Why quit eating burgers and fries only to recover and go back to a life you hated anyway? Thirty years after I recovered, I took a screenwriting course called Story, given by Robert McKee. Five years later, I audited the course and plowed through the whole three days again. Sitting in an auditorium with Bob McKee for three days reminded me of the scene in *Little Shop of Horrors* when Bill Murray is in the dentist's chair begging Steve Martin to hurt him again. The real test in a Story seminar is not whether you learn to write; it's whether you can take the verbal abuse Bob dishes out during the seminar.

Despite the abuse, I learned some good lessons. For example, for a plot or character to be good, it must have an arc. If a man starts out as a saint in chapter one, you'd better get him sinning by chapter two or you could have a one-dimensional Gumby for a character. The story needs to arc. Everything needs to change, or you don't have a story—you have a report. Second, as McKee would shout through his phlegmy cough, "Nothing is what it seems, or it better damn well not be."

If you're reading this book and you have cancer, is your goal to get rid of cancer, or have you thought about getting a whole new life? You may need a gigantic arc in your life, not just the cessation of a disease.

In 1964, I was twenty-three years old and the administrator of the New Ulm Christian School. It was an honorable job. But what I wanted to do—what I'd wanted to do my whole life—was writing and speaking—preferably comedy. I wanted to write comedy and do stand-up. But like a lot of folks, and maybe like you who are reading this, I put one foot in front of the other after high school and found myself entrenched in a life that was someone else's idea. The problem with getting well and beating cancer is that if there is no arc when we get well, we all go back to the same life we had before we got sick. For some, it isn't a great homecoming.

What I needed to do to get my *health* back was to get my *life* back. I needed a change badly, because nothing was what it seemed. About three o'clock in the afternoon, as I lay on a rug in Tijuana, I opened my mind to the possibility of major change. I could see myself doing stand-up comedy.

Steve Jobs, before his death, gave a very special speech at a Stanford University graduation about "connecting the dots." If you haven't heard it, find it on YouTube. In the speech, which was viewed by millions of people around the world in the days following his death, Jobs spoke publicly for the first time about his own possibly failing health, using that to emphasize what he told the students: "Your time is limited, so don't waste it living someone else's life . . . Have the courage to follow your heart and intuition."

Maybe someone gave you this book. Maybe you never would have selected it from a bookstore shelf. Just because you're reading this book does not necessarily mean you want to live badly enough to follow a strict program. Let me put it another way. Did you ever have a clunker car that you didn't like? Did you wash it every week? Change the oil every three thousand miles? Nope. You hated that car, so it deserved all the neglect and scorn you could heap on it. You threw McDonald's wrappers onto the backseat when you finished your bacon double cheeseburger. If you spilled a shake on the seat, you just brushed it off onto the floor, figuring it would melt. If someone opened his or her car door onto your door, who cared? We'll never take care of anything we despise. So you tell me: Why should you follow a restrictive diet if the life you have is not worth saving? May I suggest that now might be a good time to hit the reset button?

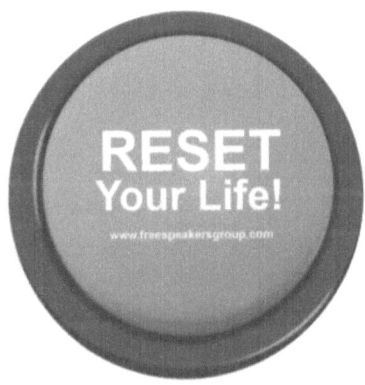

HIT THE RESET BUTTON!

At age twenty-three, I found myself living my mother's dream. Her intentions were noble and good, but she wanted me to be involved in church work, and I didn't. I woke up that day in Tijuana and realized I was a poor clone of my mom, and a horrible, Bizarro image of myself. I believe that much of my healing came from my decision that if I got well, I would pursue my life ambitions. Focusing on setting meaningful new goals rather than on getting well made me willing to make whatever sacrifices were necessary. Exactly eight years later, I did just that in Fort Lauderdale at the Comic Strip, with Sam Kinison headlining. Of course, my humor and Sam's were a tad different . . .

Some of you are in dead-end jobs that haven't made you stretch in years. Some of you are in abusive relationships. You think you deserve that idiot you married, but you don't. Some of you, if you thought you couldn't fail, would go back to school, write that great American novel, get that screenplay done, fall in love, lose fifty pounds . . . Whatever it is that you've put off for decades may indeed be part of the reason you got sick in the first place.

Try this. Place your focus beyond just getting well. Place your focus on getting excited again, the kind of excitement that makes you stay up late and get up early. The kind of excitement that makes you lose track of time. The kind of excitement in which setbacks are only a minor annoyance, because you have a laser focus that can't be compromised. Like a pimple on the butt of a prom queen, it won't matter. Woe to the disease that tries to conquer this person.

By the way, for those of you who read this book but want more information, simply log on to http://www.freespeakersgroup.com and leave your name and e-mail address so that you can listen in on free webinars, and hear about upcoming events in San Diego. Also, if you'd like a free copy of my ***Ten Strategies for Long-Term Survival after Cancer***, sign up for our mailing list and I'll send you a free copy!

My editor for this book asked me an interesting question: "What if some of the readers don't know what they want to be?" Fair question. Few of us who want to be a fireman at five years old actually grow up to be one. My only advice is to look for traits in your own life. What are you really good at? Really, now, let's be honest—most of us are really good at only one or two things. Is there an activity you do that makes time cease to exist? Is there something you do that people admire? Is there a subject that fascinates but that you haven't dedicated the time or money to learn more about? These urges are clues to your new life. Chase them, hunt them, find them, and then own them as the key to your vitality.

What if you got cancer a lot later in life than I did? What in the world does "hit the reset button" mean to a senior citizen?

Remember that I'm now sixty-one years old, so I know a little of what you may be thinking. Just this morning, I looked in the mirror when I was getting ready and said, "Dad?" After shaving my ears, I thought, *I want to make sure I address the readers who may be over sixty.* I've learned firsthand that hair on a man's body never leaves—it just relocates. I can hear the hairs talking on the top of my head:

"When ya leavin'?"

"Probably this afternoon."

"Where ya goin'?"

"Well, I thought about the ears, but then I can get only one side of things. I think, instead, I'm headed for the shoulders. That's a vantage point I can live with."

"You?"

"Oh, that's easy: the nose."

You and I need to be encouraged to hit the reset button no matter what our age might be. You may be thinking, *if I'd known about all this thirty years ago, I'd have had time to reset my life. But now, what's the point?*

Let's look at the lives of three businessmen most of you have heard of.

Ray Kroc started McDonald's in 1954 at age fifty-two. He died at eighty-two.

Dr. Forrest Shaklee started Shaklee Vitamins in 1956 at sixty-two. He died at ninety-one.

Colonel Sanders started KFC in 1956 at age sixty-six. He died at ninety.

Is it too late for you, really? And just so you don't think these guys had wealthy families who made it easy for them, remember this:

Mr. McDonald's, Ray Kroc, was a jazz piano player who sold paper cups to support his music career until he bought a restaurant from the McDonald brothers. It was no overnight success, but his net worth at his death was estimated at $1.7 billion. Not too shabby.

Dr. Shaklee lost his first business when a fire destroyed his chiropractic clinic. After starting the Shaklee Corporation, an explosion destroyed his food-supplement plant, killing some of his workers. Yet his stock at his death was worth $400 million.

Colonel Sanders went broke three times, lost two hotels, had a failed legal practice, and took restaurant-management classes before founding KFC in a gas station. His net worth at his death was $300 million.

Opportunity is abundant. Focus on doing what you're doing right now so well that you begin to love it and others couldn't do it like you even if they tried. Consider Rudyard Kipling, an English poet, short-story writer, and novelist who was born in 1865 and is chiefly remembered for his tales and poems about British soldiers in India, as well as for his tales for children. Kipling received the 1907 Nobel Prize in Literature. He wrote a short ditty that I have repeated more often than any other saying:

> *"They copied and they copied, but they couldn't copy my mind.*
> *So, I left them sweating and swearing, and a year and a half*
> *behind."*

When I made the decision to focus on getting the life I wanted, instead of on getting my health back, a wave of energy and possibility washed over me. Opportunity had been all around me for a very long time, but I just hadn't seen it.

GUIDELINES FOR HITTING
THE RESET BUTTON

It may at first glance appear that a person with a so-called "terminal" illness is at a huge disadvantage to set new goals. But let's look closer. The old adage of "never pick a fight with an ugly man because he has nothing to lose," may apply here. In October of 1974, I was on the verge of losing my life or everything. Dr. Diamandis says, ". . . with little to lose, and a passion to prove themselves, small teams [or individuals] consistently outperform large organizations when it comes to innovation." In other words, this huge crisis you are facing just may be an advantage you didn't have before. Maybe you feel like you are in a box and can't get out. Diamandis comments, "Don't think outside the box. Go box shopping. A good box is like a lane marker on the highway. It's a constraint that liberates." There will never be a time in your entire life when you are as creative as you are now. The "constraint" of possibly dying soon will focus you as never before. You may not be this much like a laser ever again.

From a practical point of view, you are probably out of money right now. The advantage in this is that whatever you do when you hit the Reset button, you will look for a way to do it economically that will make your ideas more competitive in cost. People with a ton of money and time, do not look for ways to economize and may price themselves out of any market.

The time limit a cancer person may have is another liberating constraint. Dr. Diamandis says, "In the pressure cooker of a race, with an ever-looming deadline, teams must quickly come to terms with the fact that "the same old way" won't work. So they're forced to try something new, pick a new path . . ." For all of us who have or had cancer, let's say along with Alan Kay, "The best way to predict the future is to create it!"

Here's an interesting three-way test I read in James Kunen's book, *Diary of a Company Man*—Losing a Job, Finding a Life. In this outlandish and eye-opening romp though his life, he says there are three questions to ask to make sure there is no distance between who you are and what you are doing:

- *Am I good at my work?*
- *Is it important?*
- *Am I appreciated at work and home?*

If the answers are no, time for a fresh start.

BACK TO REALITY

Within a month, my cancer markers had returned to the normal range, and I was steadily gaining weight and feeling better. The rest of the trip went according to plan, and after three weeks I was discharged as a patient with no scheduled follow-up. I now faced life in the real world as a cancer patient trying to stay well. My first startling realization that life would never be the same came on my flight home.

When Les and I boarded the plane that would take us from San Diego back to Minneapolis, I saw a familiar face in the gate area. He'd been a guest speaker at our college, so I walked over and introduced myself. He invited me to sit next to him on the flight home if we could get the person holding that seat to switch, which was easy enough. When lunch was served, I looked at my plate in horror. I turned to my friend and said, "Holy smokes! I can't eat anything on this tray, and you shouldn't, either. This stuff could kill you!"

He looked at me, looked down at his plate, looked back at me, and said, "Rick, it's a cheese sandwich."

When I walked through the door of our mobile home, I opened the kitchen cupboards and sighed. There wasn't anything in there I could eat, either. This was going to be harder than I'd thought. The first thing I did was box up all the groceries with additives, in tin cans, or with preservatives and took them to my next-door neighbor, the one we didn't really like. We were pretty sure they'd eat anything that didn't eat them first.

MOWING THE LAWN
WITH MY TEETH

I made up my mind shortly after meeting Soldier that I would do as I was told. In other words, if the doctors at the clinic told me to mow the lawn with my teeth, I'd ask them if they'd like it edged.

Sounds good, until you actually take a run at it. Old habits die hard. I hate to make you sound like a creature of habit, but I bet you eat fewer than twenty-five different foods regularly. Make a list and look in your shopping cart next time you're at the store. I bet you can tell me exactly what aisles peanut butter and jelly are in at your grocery store. Unfortunately, a lot of the foods that I was accustomed to eating were no longer on my diet sheet.

Dr. Francisco Contreras, Ernesto's son and the current director of Oasis, says, "Food is not for facial entertainment." The diet was so simple and basic that anyone could do it—but then, who would want to? The truth is, most junk food tastes great. But just so you know, here's the program I used to help me get well.

OUR FOOD BIBLE: THE LAETRILE MODIFIED DIET

The diet described below is the Laetrile modified diet, which I followed rigorously for the first five years of my recovery. To this day, I pay attention to its basic principles. It changed the way I think about food. In my opinion, the nutritional benefits from this diet were largely responsible for giving my body the chance to rebuild its natural defenses against a systemic illness like cancer.

Category	Recommended	Forbidden
BEVERAGES	Chamomile tea, clear tea, mint tea, papaya tea, Sanka	Alcohol, cocoa, coffee, soft drinks
BREAD	Rye bread, soya bread, whole-wheat or bran muffins, whole-wheat bread	White bread, all others
CEREALS	Buckwheat, cornmeal, cracked wheat, millet, oatmeal, fine-ground grits	Bleached flour, white rice, all other grains
CHEESE	Nonfat cottage cheese	All other cheeses
DESSERT	Fresh fruit, stewed fruit, gelatin	All other desserts
EGGS	Poached or boiled; limit one per day	All other forms
FAT	Cold-pressed oils, preferably safflower or corn oil	Butter, shortening, saturated oils

FISH	Very fresh white fish; only occasionally	All other fish
FRUIT	Any fresh fruit	Canned or prepared fruits
VEGETABLES	All	Canned or preserved vegetables
JUICE	Only fresh juices, mostly vegetable; fruit juice sparingly	Canned, any with additives
MEAT	Lean grilled, broiled, roasted, or baked beef, chicken, lamb, turkey, veal	Pork or any fried or fatty meats
MILK	Yogurt, buttermilk, and nonfat milk products in limited quantities	All other dairy
NUTS	All types of fresh, raw nuts	None
POTATOES	Baked, boiled, or mashed potatoes; potato salad	French fries, potato chips
SALADS	All	None
SPICES	Sea salt, chives, garlic, onion, parsley, herbs, sage, thyme,	Regular salt, pepper, paprika
SOUPS	Vegetable soup (barley, brown rice, and millet can be added)	All others
SWEETS	Unpasteurized honey, unsulphured molasses, raw sugar, carob	Candy, chocolate, white sugar

Any variation in this diet should be done only with a doctor's permission. Avoid all toxic materials, including smoking and other forms of tobacco. Keep away from secondhand smoke.

Clearly, new dietary information has come to light since this diet was printed. For example, this diet forbids coffee, but new studies have shown coffee to be a very effective antioxidant. Dark chocolate (in moderation and with at least 60 percent cocoa) is fine in moderation. New sweeteners like Stevia and Agave make coffee drinkable again. Add a dash of Silk soy milk and you have a Starbucks-quality creation.

Diet remains the trickiest part of an ongoing program. Anyone can be a hero for a day, but being diligent for thirty-eight years is impossible. However, if you have cancer and I can convince you to be mostly a hero for five years, you just may do very well. If you hang in there for five, you'll wind up with a much healthier diet than if you'd done it for only a few weeks.

DETOXIFICATION, SUPPLEMENTATION, AFFIRMATION

I wish the story could end here—happy endings are nice, huh? It would have been great if I'd gotten well and then returned home to become rich and famous. As my systematic theology professor said one day after one of my thornier questions, "Yeah, well, real life is messy."

At this point in the story, the rubber meets the road. You can get caught up in the battle and forget that real life goes on. I faced a bit of a letdown when I got home and realized that I now had to follow this boring diet for . . . the rest of my life. Really? Once I got home, no one would be flying into town to check on me. I wouldn't be having high-level talks with Mayo Clinic doctors. Gone were the people who gathered in the lobby daily to fight for their lives. Tomorrow morning would come, and Frosted Flakes were out. No baloney sandwich for lunch or McDonald's for dinner. It was way more fun planning to change my life than actually changing it. But if this book is going to be a real resource, it needs to relay information not only on how I got well but how I stayed well. Could it be that people who do chemotherapy or radiation have some degree of post-traumatic stress disorder? When patients start to get well, and people stop coming around, it's back to real life, but no one's paying attention. Hardcore soldiers have trouble living routine lives.

I've already spilled the beans (no pun intended) about colonics, but let me add that it never occurred to me that this would be a weekly part of my life for five solid years.

Here's the drill: Sunday afternoon would be my last meal for three days. I'd go to the store and buy four or five watermelons. In the winter, the cashiers gave me the weirdest looks, because I was paying ten dollars for each small melon. The glycemic index is pretty high on watermelons, and folks with active cancer and tumors need to limit that sugar. But watermelons are also very alkaline. Plus, the sugar in watermelons made it possible for me to do three days of fasting without getting the shakes and big-time headaches associated with water fasts. I'd haul the old Champion juicer out (I burned out two of them), cut the ends off the melons, and chuck them. Then I'd slice the melon into strips that would fit through the juicer, rind and all; keep in mind that I had cut the ends off and didn't try to juice all that rind. But a little rind makes the juice more refreshing, giving it a hint of cucumber flavor. I'd drink six to eight ounces and refrigerate the rest in a sealed pitcher. Every two to three hours, I'd have another glass. Have you ever wanted more time in a day? Try fasting. Time drags by at a snail's pace. You start watching the clock for your next "fix" of juice.

By nighttime on the first day, my energy would be gone. Before bed, I'd eat a big slice of watermelon, because it would trick my body into thinking it had gotten something to eat—and I could sleep. Otherwise I'd lie awake, thinking, *What in this room could I trade for a steak and fries?* I heard a speaker once claim he'd given up bad food and never wanted it again. Really? Come on. Not me. I never stopped thinking about fries and BLTs. I thought about them as often two years into my program as I did prior to starting the program.

By the next morning, my stomach had shrunk enough so I wasn't really hungry when I got out of bed. I'd open the refrigerator and stare at all the food. Then I'd walk to the cupboard and open it, just trying to get a glimpse of what I wouldn't be eating that day. Finally I'd reopen the fridge, grab my pitcher of juice, and pour a glass while thinking, *Hey, another day, another glass.* I'd also take some herbal laxatives with Cascara Sagrada or Senna to clean the pipes. By the third day, I was so cleaned out, I squeaked when I walked.

On Wednesday night, I'd do my homemade colonic. I bought a hot-water bottle and syringe. Usually these are advertised for feminine douching, which, of course, I didn't do much. The hose has a clip for controlling the flow of water. You can either hang the water bottle on the shower rod or hold it. I'd lie down on a towel, elevate my feet, and, well, you get it by now.

I welcomed Thursday morning, because at that point I could eat some fruit or oatmeal. Real food! The big surprise was that digesting food takes energy, and I'd often feel like a nap after breakfast (which actually means "break the fast"). For a period of five years, I ate solid food only from Thursday through Sunday afternoon. The rest of the time, I fasted. Was this too extreme? Maybe. I just didn't want to test the theory by not doing it.

The Laetrile modified diet allowed me to eat things like organic chicken a couple of times a week, homemade soups, and almost any kind of vegetables. Once in a while I'd splurge and try handmade pizza (no pepperoni) or some venison, if we could get it. I limited sugar in my diet and drank no soda pop. I drank no alcohol (but about halfway through the fourth year, I had a glass of wine and nearly fell down). To illustrate just how detoxed you can get, we took a trip to the Hippocrates Health Institute about a year after I'd been to Oasis. Hippocrates was in Boston at that time but currently it's in West Palm Beach, Florida. For almost a month, we ate nothing but watermelon, a wheatberry juice called Rejuvilac, and sprout salads. Just before it was time to leave, we snuck out to the No Name fish restaurant, and I ordered some grilled halibut and potatoes. Just before dinner was over, I started drinking more and more water, until I had a thirst stronger than any thirst I had ever had. Apparently I had been eating so little salt that when I ate the salted fish and potatoes, my body really reacted. I was also up half the night "detoxing." Hippocrates was like another planet. The owner, Ann Wigmore, was a piece of work, to say the least. She walked around with a miniature monkey on her shoulder and talked about offering classes on colonics. I wasn't about to drop my lily whites in front of a lot of left-of-center folks and teach them where to stick the hose.

We met people who said they were "airtarians," which meant they didn't eat or drink at all; they just lived off the energy of the universe . . . like ferns. We met vegetarians, fruitarians, vegans, and some who looked like they'd been dead for several years. I guess any discipline attracts extremists.

I faintly remember that when I was a small child, my grandmother took something that looked like a turkey baster, sat us in the sink, and administered what I would call a mini-colonic. Country folks had their own natural remedies for anything, and colonics made perfect sense to them. One day just a few weeks ago, I wasn't feeling well, so I gathered my colonic equipment and headed to the bathroom. My daughter, Heather, saw me walk by and casually said, "Not feeling well, Dad?" My family associates colonics with healing.

If you asked me what made long-term health possible for me after cancer, I would say it was mostly having an ongoing detox program.

You have to enjoy life as much as possible during your recovery. I accomplished this through creative cheating. About once a week, I would look forward to eating something that I wouldn't normally eat, as a treat. It wasn't something toxic, but it also wasn't on my diet. I'd usually indulge on Sunday, before the fast began. My favorite treat was a grilled peanut butter and jelly sandwich. I'd get organic butter, bread, peanut butter, and jelly and grill the sandwich like a grilled cheese. I can't tell you how good that tasted after a solid week of watermelon juice. Also on Sundays, we'd broil a small piece of chicken or fish for our Sunday dinner. Dark chocolate was a treat I let myself have about once a month. I didn't eat a five-pound block, just enough so I knew I was standing there munching on chocolate like a real person.

One time, when I was lecturing on my diet after returning from Mexico, a woman raised her hand and said, "You make it sound like if we ever go to McDonald's, we won't go to heaven." Everyone chuckled, and I answered, "No, eating at McDonald's won't keep you out of heaven. In fact, I think you'll get there quicker."

In case you still think I goofed by leaving the Mayo Clinic, consider the fact that my first meal when I came out of surgery was Jell-O and 7UP. This meal probably contained five tablespoons of white sugar, which, by the way, tasted great.

Food allergies were not a consideration back in 1974, but today, thankfully, they are. If you have a history of headaches and digestion problems like bloating, gas, or diarrhea/constipation, you may want to take some food allergy tests, especially concerning dairy, wheat, corn, and soy.

Even when I was coming off a fast and eating all-natural foods, my headaches remained pretty constant until I was fifty-five years old. Now, at sixty-one years old, headaches are a distant memory—ever since I got off gluten. Gluten-free food is now available in nearly all health-food stores and even in larger grocery stores. Many restaurants cater to gluten allergies and have a gluten-free menu. Some restaurants, such as Hooleys in Rancho San Diego, offer many of their menu items in gluten-allergy-friendly form. Eddie, the barkeep, is up on what ingredients are in the food and is always watching out for his patrons.

Support and information groups are available, such as The Celiac Sprue Association http://www.csaceliacs.info, a national support organization that provides information and referral services for persons with celiac disease. Blood tests are available, but when I attended a gluten-free meeting organized by Meetup.com, I heard a lot of people say they got a false negative on their blood test. Most don't want to submit to a biopsy. My blood tests, which were taken on November 15, 2004, at South County Hospital in Wakefield, Rhode Island, showed the following out-of-range values:

Test name	Out of range	Normal range
Antigliadin Ab,IgG	103	0-19 units
Antigliadin Ab, IgA	136	0-19 units
Tissue Transglutaminase	175	0-19 units

Whatever your food allergy turns out to be, if you have one at all, muster up the discipline to get off those foods and stay off. Your allergic reaction may very well be suppressing your immune system—and we both know what that can do.

The day you return home after trying an alternative treatment, expect Murphy's Law to be in force (whatever can go wrong, will go wrong, at the worst possible time). Why friends and family think they need to straighten you out now that you've gotten that "Mexican thing" out of your system, I'll never know. They start giving you the names of *real* doctors, or the best doctors. They invite you out for hot dogs and beer to get your system back to normal. They go online and start telling you about people who went south of the border and never came back. But my personal favorite is when they walk up, take your wilted hand in theirs, furrow their brow, and ask, "How are you doing? I mean, really?"

The implication is crystal clear: you're toast, and you should admit it. Squeeze their hand until it turns blue and then yank your hand back and shout, "If I were any better, you could bottle me." Get out of bed every day and get on the path to your new life. Don't lie in bed unless you're prevented from leaving it. Take a shower, look your best, and start taking steps that will lead you to the life you seek. Act like it's already here—it's just hiding. Don't poll the people in your life about the economy, politics, or the state of existence. Tell them what you believe about good health. The ones on your team will encourage you. The ones with a hidden agenda will stop coming around. You're in charge of this new life, and if anyone tries to get you off your diet or distract you from your goals—get new friends. I mean it! I'm not encouraging you to dump your husband or wife, but if your spouse poisons your mind or your efforts (mine did not), at least limit their opportunities to get you down. It's your life, and you need to start protecting it. Believe me, people will start to leave you when you're no longer a footstool. Stand tall, look them right in the eye, and say what's in your heart.

I was standing at the sink one morning, drinking a green drink and taking about forty supplements. My father was visiting, and after watching me for a few seconds, he said in his southern drawl, "Well, I'll swear, why would anyone eat that many pills?"

I wheeled around, looked him right in the eye, and said in a very loud, direct voice, "It beats chemotherapy." I held his eyes and would not look away.

That was the last comment he made.

When you get home from a place like Oasis of Hope, all the toxic, bad foods you left behind will be waiting for you like a band of terrorists. *Before taking off your coat*, grab a large box and fill it with canned goods, anything with preservatives, sugary anything—gather everything not on your diet and put it in the box. Lock the box(es) in the trunk of your car and take them to a shelter for homeless people. They would rather have toxic food than no food. I would, too.

Do not let others grocery shop for you. I don't care if grocery shopping ranks right up there with a root canal; you do it so that you and you alone are responsible for the kind of food in that house. Here's the truth: if it's bad for you, and it's in the house, you will eat it. Sooner or later, you'll walk in your sleep and find that Snickers bar hidden behind the juicer. Do you know how I know this? I own a juicer, of course.

You'll get invited to dinner at friends' houses. Just to prove they're really your friends, they'll serve pork chops smothered in gravy, followed by chocolate cake for dessert. Thank them and tell them you had a late lunch, but if they'll let you make a salad, you're all set. People should no longer dictate to you what you will and will not eat or do. Here's the best approach: when you are invited for a meal, politely tell your hosts that you are now on a very restrictive diet, and outline what you can and cannot eat. If you were a smoker, every smoker on the planet will offer you a smoke—right after dinner, when you want it most. If you take that cigarette, you're sending your body a mixed signal. When you got on your new diet, your body probably thought, *Good deal! This person cares if I live or die, and the stuff he's giving me now is making a difference.* If you take that cigarette, your body will think, *Say what? What did I do wrong? Now you're trying to kill me.*

Think I'm kidding? Nope. It's scientific. Dr. William H. Frey II, a biochemist at the St. Paul-Ramsey Medical Center in Minnesota, measured the chemical content of tears in different situations. He and his team analyzed two types of tears: emotional tears (from crying when emotionally upset and stressed) and tears arising from irritants (such as crying from cutting onions). They found that emotional tears contained more of the protein-based hormones prolactin, adrenocorticotropic hormone, and leucine enkephalin (a natural painkiller), all of which are produced by the body when it's under stress. It seems as if the body is getting rid of these chemicals through tears.

Go back to work as soon as you can, or start building that lifelong dream business. Get back in the game. Time spent worrying about your cancer is time wasted. Every time I got the slightest pain, I was sure it was my cancer spreading. Put those thoughts out of your mind, or at least stop them once they start. If a friend starts relating a long, gory story about someone who just died from your kind of cancer, stop him or her mid-sentence and say, "I know you're trying to be helpful, but right now listening to a story about a cancer death is not helping me." I could write two more chapters about the nutty, insensitive things people did and said to me when I got home. After I returned to work at the Christian School, I spoke one Sunday night about what the Bible says about food. The next day, one of the kids who'd heard me speak marched up, opened his lunchbox, and shouted, "Thanks for nothing! Look what my mom packed today for lunch!" I saw an apple, a bag of carrot sticks, and an avocado-and-sprout sandwich. I'm pretty sure he trashed most of it at lunch. Some members of your family will never eat like you're eating, though it would be nice if they did. My wife put the whole family on the diet. My daughter, Heather, put no processed or toxic food in her mouth until she went to school. We'd seat her in the highchair and put alfalfa sprouts on her tray. She'd reach over and munch them like a cow chewing cud. Too cute, huh?

If your family refuses to help, eat at a different time. You can't be expected to sit there crunching bean sprouts while your significant other gorges on a double cheeseburger and fries and washes it all down with a Coke. Of course, you could slap him or her upside the head, grab the burger and fries, and throw them out the front door . . . or not.

If you used to smoke, avoid going places where people smoke. If you used to have a cocktail or five after work, don't go to the bar. Instead, go to the local juice bar and order an orange juice. If you go to that bar, it'll be only a matter of time before your orange juice is 50 percent vodka, and you know it. If sweets were your thing, don't stop at Krispy Kreme just because the "Ready Now" light is on. I'm ragging on you, because the first few weeks after you dedicate yourself to a new kind of life will be when you're tested the most. I want you to be able to say, "I'm happy I did" instead of "I wish I had."

I stayed on the very restrictive diet for at least five years. Then I slowly allowed myself to drift back toward a more traditional diet without the toxic foods. For example, I eat red meat about once a week, but I try to get meat raised without chemicals. I allow myself to enjoy a glass of red wine with a good dinner or a gluten-free beer with gluten-free pizza. But staying on a very strict program for five years allowed my immune system to rebuild, and, in my opinion, this is the basis of long-term survival.

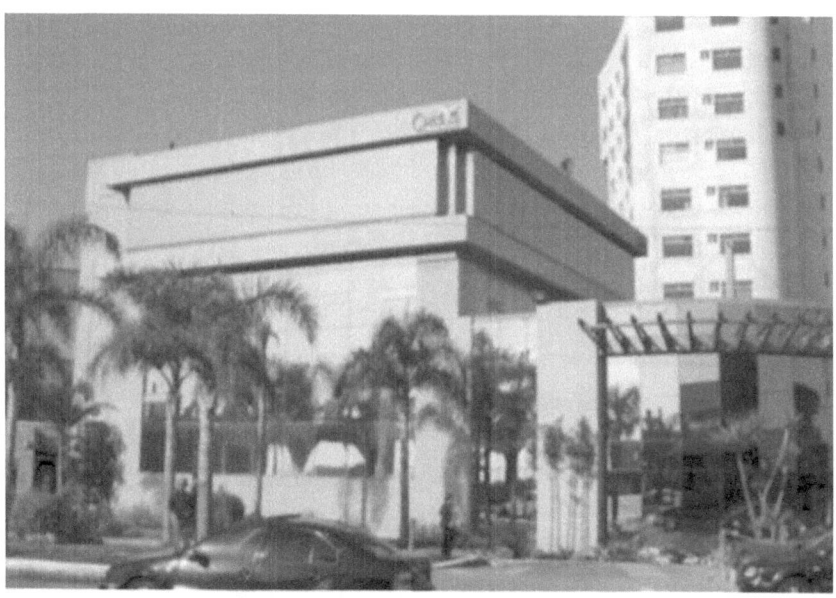

The Oasis of Hope hospital as it looks today, not as it looked in 1974.

Getting well and knowing how you got well are two different things. There were so many of us in Tijuana back in 1974 that personal attention was difficult for the staff to provide. We really didn't know why the treatment was supposed to work, but desperate people will try a lot of things.

Since moving to San Diego in 2011, I've had the opportunity to attend some lectures at the Oasis of Hope Hospital and discover why what I did actually worked. I've told you what it was like to be there in the early seventies, but now let me tell you what it's like when I visit to attend a lecture or have lunch. It's been fascinating and reinforcing for me to learn about the science behind what I did in the seventies. There wasn't time for lectures or Q&A sessions back then, but today, the doctors teach you how the program works in your body and what is happening that can make you well.

I get on the 805 South around ten o'clock on Wednesday morning and drive to the last exit before the border. I choose one of the parking lots that charge about seven dollars a day. After parking the car, I walk into Mexico, and it's nothing like entering the States. There is never a line, never a wait. Drug-sniffing dogs approach and sniff your bags, if you have any, but that's it. I walk to the McDonald's located two minutes from the border, and Oasis picks me up in a nice van. The ride to the hospital—which is still located across the street from the ocean-side bullring—takes about ten minutes. You can easily see downtown San Diego and the Coronado Bridge from the hillside; it is quiet, safe, and very picturesque. The van drops me off at the front door, and I'm always impressed by the design of this modern five-story structure. Inside, I'm greeted at the front desk, and then I turn left into a large, well-appointed cafeteria. I love to eat there; all the food is on my diet, it's prepared correctly, and it actually tastes good. Fresh-squeezed juices are always available. Just before noon, the patients eating in the cafeteria and I go to the third floor and pass many patient rooms, which are nicely decorated and cheery, with lots of natural light. The activity room usually seats about twenty-five patients and guests. When Dr. Francisco Contreras enters the room, all goes quiet. He's handsome like his father was and has that totally engaging Contreras smile. He's trim and usually dresses casually in jeans and a jacket. For the next hour or so, he explains why the program works. Most hospitals dispense medicines without explaining the mechanics of how your body will use them. Doctors at the Oasis of Hope Hospital not only explain but also stick around to answer questions.

One morning, as I waited in the hallway to go into Dr. Contreras' lecture, Mary Bernal, Dr. Contreras's assistant, approached and pointed down the hallway. "Rick, see that woman standing at the end of the hall, talking to some patients?" she asked. I looked and nodded. "She was here about the same time you were—go talk to her."

"What?" I said, grinning. "I thought I was the oldest living relic from the original Good Samaritan Clinic."

I found Betty Couty talking to some folks and introduced myself. Of course, she was as happy to find me as I was to find her. Nothing is more encouraging than meeting someone who has had good success, especially from thirty-eight years ago. Betty was literally carried into the clinic back in April of 1975 with stage-four cancer. Today, she lives in Fort Lauderdale and is busy with her grandkids.

I'm going to give you my take on why the program works, based on my experience and the notes I took during some of Dr. Francisco's lectures. I make no claim that I heard all of it correctly, but I think I remember enough of it to make sense. However, keep in mind that at my age, memory is the second thing to go.

FEED, STARVE, BUILD

Breaking this down into a simple, memorable formula may help us keep doing the basics. I once asked a friend who was very successful in the vitamin business how he became the number-one distributor. He paused for a moment, and then, with a straight face, he said, "Stop doing the wrong things, and start doing the right things."

I felt like saying, "Thanks, Obi-Won, but I was looking for a little more content." But you know what? Thirty-eight years later, I understand that being healthy really is about stopping harmful things and starting healthy things.

Cancer cells and tumors hate an oxygen-rich environment. The less oxygen a tumor has, the more aggressive it becomes. So why not just jump into an oxygen tent? Because breathing pure oxygen can be addictive and even fatal.

Tumors hate oxygen—a fact otherwise called tumor hypoxia. According to Wikipedia: "Tumor hypoxia is the situation where tumor cells have been deprived of oxygen. As a tumor grows, it rapidly outgrows its blood supply, leaving portions of the tumor with regions where the oxygen concentration is significantly lower than in healthy tissues."

Hypoxic tumor cells are usually resistant to radiotherapy and chemotherapy, but they can be made more susceptible to treatment by if you increase the amount of oxygen in them. Even chemo won't work as well if the tumor has become hypoxic. So how do you get more oxygen to a tumor so that chemo and other modalities can work?

Ozone-treated blood has proven to be very effective. In 2004, Dr. Bernardino Clavo of Spain (MD, PhD Oncology) published papers concerning the efficacy of taking about 300 ccs of blood out of a patient, ozonating it, and replacing it in the patient's body. Small clinics sprang up all over the States using this method, but the FDA quickly shut them down. Red blood cells are often too large to effectively penetrate a hypoxic tumor. The Russians developed an artificial blood called Perftec, whose oxygen-delivering molecules are a hundred times smaller than those in red blood cells. Ozonate Perftec, introduce it to the blood supply, and watch tumors begin to shrink.

Nutrients and Supplements

Nutrients are the signal to the cells in a process called signal transduction. When we eat a lot of fresh, organic vegetables and a smaller amount of fruits, we send the right signals to the cells. Food supplements are designed to send larger signals than food. It's important to take them religiously, especially for the first five years. Oasis suggests large doses of vitamin C, for instance. In the 1970s, Dr. Linus Pauling was the first to use nutrients as a drug in the treatment of disease. His papers on vitamin C were revolutionary, and he coined the term "nutraceuticals." Dr. Mark Levine discovered that very high doses (4 grams per kilo of body weight) of ascorbic acid (vitamin C) reduced tumors in mice up to 50 percent.

Shark cartilage offers some promise as a supplement and has been used at Oasis with success. In 1983, two researchers at the Massachusetts Institute of Technology published a study showing that shark cartilage contains a substance that significantly inhibits the development of blood vessels that nourish solid tumors, thereby limiting tumor growth.

Working independently, medical researchers at Harvard University Medical School found that if one could inhibit angiogenesis—the development of a new blood network—one could prevent the development of tumor-based cancer and metastasis.

I'd estimate that I have spent at least $40,000 on food supplements since I left Oasis. I'm sure I've given at least $30,000 of that to purchase Shaklee nutrition. Over the years, companies like Shaklee have produced some of the finest supplements available. Before the advent of the Internet and mass spectrometry, companies thrived by announcing a secret ingredient that was known only to them. Usually they told an entertaining story about a far-flung scientist, well over a hundred years old, who'd accidentally stumbled upon a strange and wonderful plant deep in the Amazon. Luckily for us, hundreds of miles of this wonderful plant populated this remote region. Skillfully, using stainless-steel tongs under the light of a full moon, this scientist extracted a few specimens and brought them back to Harvard Medical School, where extensive testing showed the plant to be an antioxidant without equal that works at the cellular level. (Every time I hear someone say, "It works at the cellular level," my sphincter tightens and I zone out.)

According to these stories, Dr. Schmots and his crack team of researchers immediately headed back and organized an army of very small people who'd never before seen white people to carefully harvest these plants under the strictest conditions. Then they posed for PR photos wearing only large Band-Aid-type coverings.

Whenever you hear about a secret ingredient, Google it. I can just about guarantee that it's currently being sold in at least five countries—usually outside the reach of our FDA and FTC. With modern technology, it can be analyzed and synthesized in less than a month. Personally, I'm glad to see the folklore fade away. Better technology has leveled the playing field and made nutritional science more reliable—though, admittedly, not as much fun. Let's not be overly harsh on the nutritional charlatans. How many charlatans have there been in medicine over the years? How many people needlessly die on operating tables every year? How many hospital patients die from drug errors? How many die from MRSA and other bacterial or viral infections in hospitals? Still, we all want the science of nutrition to advance and remain free of excess government restrictions—and charlatans.

Nutrition is not the only area of focus for someone in recovery. Drinking pure water is essential. Personally, I like filtration at the faucet, because with whole-house systems of water purification, contamination of the giant filter or contamination in the delivery pipes can occur. Today's technology delivers really good filtration with even Brita-type pitchers. Some filter pitchers even claim to remove microbials. Clearly, drink filtered water that you control. Most bottled water is just tap water. Google "Penn & Teller: The Truth about Bottled Water"—it's hysterical and spot on, although be aware, their language can get a bit graphic. Shower filters are a great idea because tests show that we inhale ten times more chlorine by taking a hot ten-minute shower than we do by drinking chlorinated water.

We started drinking purified tap water with a giant water distiller about the size of a small Volkswagen. From that, we started drinking water that's filtered at the tap with all kinds of reverse osmosis and UV light gadgets. The newest innovation is to drink ionized water or water that has been made more alkaline through electrolysis. I own a Tyent unit (http://www.tyentusa.com) and drink alkaline water. Interestingly enough, the anti-oxidant level of this water is off the charts!

Many people buy good organic food when they are on a health program, then take the food home and cook it to death. Personally, I use Professional Platinum Cooking Systems™ (http://www.platinumcookware.com). Should you contact them, mention my book and we will contribute $25 to the Oasis hospital. Because their grade of stainless steel uses high levels of chromium oxide, it resists staining and pitting. I like it because it has even heat distribution, and the ability to cook food properly near 185 degrees with little-to-no water or oils. Additionally, we plan on hosting cooking classes on our website. Food prep is a key to long-term recovery.

Another key area for health is the air we breathe. I'm currently running four air purifiers in a three-thousand-square-foot home. I prefer zone purification over in-duct units, because the rooms farthest away from the purifier are usually not evenly purified. For years I've been a pitchman for Healthy Perceptions (http://healthyperceptions.com) because they sell a three-pack of zone air purifiers that travel well and work well in a home.

Those who take health seriously get regular Chiropractic care. Personally, wherever I live, I log on to *Activator Methods* (www.activatormethods.com) and find an *advanced proficiency*-rated Activator chiropractor in my area. I traveled and spoke for Dr. Arlan Fuhr and have seen only Activator doctors for the last fifteen years for my personal adjustments. I am aware that some chiropractors and D.O.s simply buy an Activator tool and go to work without proper training. Only those doctors trained personally by Activator Methods get regular visits from me.

When we visit the Oasis of Hope Hospital, we are visiting nutritional royalty. The history of alternative (now known as integrative) medicine started in the thirties with Dr. Otto Warburg. He won a Nobel Prize for showing that tumors require a low-oxygen environment to flourish. But it was Dr. Max Gerson, Dr. Joseph M. Issels, and Dr. Ernesto Contreras who took the information from Warburg, Pauling, and others and actually began to use it in cancer treatment. They endured investigations by government agencies and long interviews that forced them to defend their right to use safe and effective natural means. All integrative medicine today stands on the shoulders of these pioneering doctors who showed the world that profit was not the only consideration when medical care was being administered.

Starve Tumors

Tumors need protein to survive. The mechanism is NF-kappa B. There are naturally occurring NF-kappa B inhibitors like resveratrol. NF-kappa B produces white blood cells and gives tumor cells a "nonexpiration date" for survival. Tumors simply do not die if they are given enough NF-kappa B.

Tumors need insulin (sugar) to survive. High-glycemic foods increase the production of insulin, which is good for tumors. We should eat foods that are less than 70 percent on the glycemic index.

These last two paragraphs may sound scholarly, but let me once again get the crackers and peanut butter down to a shelf where you can reach them. If protein and sugar are good for tumors and bad for you, the implications for what we can and cannot eat are fairly clear, right?

Most of us like meat. We are both carnivores and omnivores. We have sharp incisors, our eyes are in front for hunting, our digestive system produces bile, and we have claws—even if we do keep them neatly trimmed. In my opinion, we were designed to eat meat. But when our immune system gets depressed and cancer proliferates, this kind of protein is not good.

It never failed. Around the third day of my fast, I'd see a Burger King commercial featuring a thick, juicy patty tumbling onto a flaming grill. This perfect patty was then lovingly placed on a toasted sesame-seed bun with pickles, tomatoes, lettuce, and mayo. A voiccover asked, "Aren't you hungry? Want it your way?" I remember looking at the TV with tears in my eyes, saying, "Yes! Yes, I want it my way—any way—just give it to me!" Sometimes my next-door neighbor grilled steaks. There they were, sizzling on the grill, smoke pouring off those bad boys into my yard and up my nose. A pot of corn on the cob boiled on a burner next to the steaks, and the picnic table was all set. I wanted to lean over the fence and offer a year's worth of slave labor for a seat at the table. Oh, and fried chicken? My mother used to get out her iron skillet, float a mountain of lard in it, and fry chicken *slowly*. She did almost twenty minutes per side to make it extra crispy. Then, when the chicken was done, she'd drain most of the grease out and leave the cracklins. Next she'd sprinkle white flour in the skillet and, with a fork, start stirring the roux while adding milk. Once she had right consistency for gravy, she'd add lots of black pepper. This was the milk gravy we dumped over potatoes, white bread, and anything else we could slop it on. Her chicken would crunch with every bite. Stop eating that protein? Are you insane?

But the one meat that should be protected under the Federal Witness Protection Program is ring bologna fried in an iron skillet with ketchup smothered on top. I mean the kind of bologna that bubbles up in the middle and burns on the edges. Slap that baby on some Wonder Bread, hit it again with the ketchup, and you're good to go. Mom also made fried Spam sandwiches, even though the ingredients of Spam are sealed in a vault somewhere near Paducah. My father was a ship's navigator in World War II, my mother, a WAVE. They lived on Spam. Winston Churchill said that outside of the Allied forces, Spam did as much to win the war as anything. It kept our far-flung troops from starving; whatever it's made of, it can survive a nuclear winter. You can't hurt it. Bullets won't go through the can. Stack them up and use them for chairs and tables. Throw them in the air for target practice. I'm not promoting Spam, but if I were in a trench, surrounded by the enemy for days or weeks, and all I had to eat was Spam—would I eat it? All I could open in one sitting. But clearly, given the option of better food, leave the Spam, bologna, fried chicken, and even T-bones alone until you're well enough (five years?) to add them slowly and sparingly back into your diet. The bologna and Spam might be better left out for good, and any meat you do eat, try to get organic, grass-raised if possible. Today, local buying clubs are popping up all over the country. Google "organic meats" and your city, and you might just find a local buying club or farm near you.

Sugar is a harder problem than protein, because the average American eats 160 pounds of sugar a year. Picture a ten-pound bag of sugar. Now pile sixteen of them up. Then grab a spoon, open the first bag, and start eating. You couldn't eat even one ten-pound bag without getting sick, but you manage to eat sixteen bags a year because sugar is hidden in almost everything we eat. We've all heard about the sugar content of Coke, cereals, and ketchup. How much is there? One teaspoon of granulated sugar equals 4 grams of sugar. Put another way, 16 grams of sugar in a product is equal to about four teaspoons of granulated sugar. How about bottled spaghetti sauce at 12 grams of sugar? How about 50 grams of sugar in some bottled teas? Lemonade purported to be 100 percent natural—30 grams. It's in everything. And now we have to learn glycemic indexes of foods. It may be a good idea to Google "low-glycemic foods" and print out a list. Even better, search for "low-glycemic desserts or snacks"—they're the things that really knock us out. In 1900, the average American consumed about ninety pounds of sugar a year. Today, he or she eats seventy pounds *more* a year. Eeeewwww.

Have I made the case for consuming a very small amount of proteins and sugars? We haven't even touched on buying only organic brands. Thankfully, even large grocery chains like Vons in California carry their O (for organic) brands. When you try to buy a product, you'll usually find an organic alternative under their O brand—so choose wisely. Producers of processed foods would stop adding harmful chemicals if we quit buying those foods. Every time we reach for an organic brand, we vote with our dollars. Follow the money trail; it will succeed every time.

Build the Immune System

I saved this one for last, because it is really the combination of everything we've discussed so far: it's the blending of a healthy mind, body, and spirit. A lot has been written about self-esteem over the years, from Wayne Dyer's *I'm Okay, You're Okay*, to the hilarious Al Franken (now the junior senator from Minnesota) as Stuart Smalley on *Saturday Night Live*:

> **Announcer**: "Daily Affirmation with Stuart Smalley." Stuart Smalley is a caring nurturer, a member of several twelve-step programs, but not a licensed therapist.
> **Stuart Smalley**: Because I'm good enough, I'm smart enough, and, doggonit, people like me!

During the seventies, gigantic positive mental attitude (PMA) rallies were held all over America, with speakers like Zig Ziglar, Paul Harvey, Dennis Waitley, Robert Shuler, W. Clement Stone, Art Linkletter, Norman Vincent Peale, Jim Rohn, Earl Nightingale, and Og Mandino. I've personally been speaking on the platform with Ziglar, Shuler, and Mandino.

Then came the "fire walks" with Anthony Robbins. Anthony Robbins is known for his bestselling books *Unlimited Power* and *Awaken the Giant Within*, Personal Power infomercials, and fire-walking seminars, as well as for being one of the foremost experts in personal change. Much of his early success was attributed to his knowledge and use of neuro-linguistic programming (NLP).

I was having a glass of wine at Club Boca in 1985 when a woman came up to me, gushing. She had just been to an Anthony Robbins fire walk, and she had succeeded.

"So," I said, "you actually walked on a bed of hot coals today?"

"I did!" she nearly shouted. "And once you do that, you can do anything!" Sally Jesse Raphael, a popular talk-show host in the eighties, was standing next to me, and she leaned in to better hear the conversation.

About a minute later, the firewalker lit a cigarette (you could smoke indoors back then). I couldn't help myself; I had to go for the joke. "Been smoking a long time?" I asked.

"Yes, since I was about twenty. I'd like to quit, but I just can't."

The disconnect, of course, is obvious. She can walk on fire, but she can't keep from sticking something on fire in her mouth. Still, we can all agree on one thing: our attitude determines most of what we think and do, which determines our outcome to a great extent.

Who among us grew up in Disneyland? Who had two perfect parents, a house with clean sheets every week on every bed? Who among us woke to find our mother lovingly placing perfectly ironed clothes at the foot of the bed? Who came home from school, found milk and cookies on the table, and heard, "Go out and play; dinner will be ready in one hour"? If you did, you're in the minority. Most of us slugged it out growing up. We did our own laundry, cooked a lot of our own meals, and lied to people who came to the front door to keep them from shutting off our utilities. Most of us were lied to, stolen from, and pounded into submission—and that's only family so far. Who among us had too much love?

Is it any wonder that so many people grow up feeling like a pair of brown shoes in a room full of tuxedos? After quickly reviewing my GPA, my high-school guidance counselor told me that I should get a good spot on the line (near a fan at a punch-press factory). In high school, I had a stutter and stood at four feet eleven—so you can quickly see why those Nightingale tapes floored me. Succeed? At what? How? Later, thrown into a battle for my life, why would I think I could win that battle?

When you feel your life is not enough, that you're doing unimportant things, and that you're always in a rush, it's difficult to have and maintain vibrant health. These are the issues that I needed to address and conquer to stop a terminal illness. Perhaps these are areas of concern for you.

I developed three affirmations that I used like mantras. I repeated these to myself several times a day to offset my knee-jerk belief that I was worthy of a long, horrible death. Here they are:

1. **I AM ENOUGH**—I'm tall enough, smart enough, and tough enough to get through this. Everything I need to be free of this disease I already have. I need only to embrace it and not waiver.

2. **I HAVE TIME**—Around two in the afternoon, have you ever found yourself with your shoulders hunched up to your ears, head pounding, fretting about one thing or another? The ability to relax and pursue your new goals with quiet confidence gives you great power that others just don't use. When we're at work, we feel guilty that we're not home with the kids. When we're with the kids, we worry about the work piling up. We're really never anywhere in this state of mind. Eleanor Roosevelt said it best when she said, "Yesterday is history. Tomorrow is a mystery. Today is a gift; that's why it is called the present."

3. **WHAT I DO IS IMPORTANT**—Ever lie down at night and wonder what the heck you did all day? Once we get all the financial holes filled in and have the necessities and some of the niceties of life, we need to find meaning in what we do. For most of us, meaning comes from our work. Make no mistake: according to the psychologist William James, most of our reward in life comes not from leisure but from work. When you hit the reset button, did you hit it hard enough? Did you decide to attempt something important? Are people depending on you to succeed? Or could you walk off the end of a dock without anyone noticing? Writing this book is important, because over the years, other editions of it have provided hope and a few chuckles. It's rewarding to hear from readers that they started a new and exciting life after having read my books. I just wish I could meet that high-school counselor again someday that thought my greatest potential was to stand near a fan in the factory.

LIFE AFTER HITTING
THE RESET BUTTON

It was a chilly, windy day on the beach in Tijuana when I made the decision to reset my life. What happened in the next few years was a whirlwind of opportunity rooted in an astonishing amount of available energy. Think back over your life and identify the really productive years. How many years were magic? When did you make great strides in creating the life you wanted? The next few pages detail the wild and wacky way I found huge opportunities once I opened my mind to possibilities.

In 1975, I was attending Cornerstone University's graduate program (then called Grand Rapids Theological Seminary). I was working in a shoe store part time and my wife was giving piano lessons on an upright piano we bought for $50 and spray painted blue. We had signed up to buy Shaklee vitamins before leaving Minnesota and slowly I started telling people about my gigantic health change using nutrition in Mexico. Less than a year later, we were driving a new company car and vacationing in London rather than Detroit.

One day, a visiting pastor spoke in chapel and said he was concerned about a trend at the school. He said that young men were not trusting the Lord for their support but were instead starting businesses "just in case" the ministry didn't pan out. He glared directly at me during his remarks.

I went home that day and asked my wife if she really cared if I graduated. She said no, and I never went back, not even to say goodbye. What really bothered me was that if I had failed in my business, no one would have cared. If I had just done so-so, there would have been no complaints. But because I was making more money than the school's president, I was suspect. In other words, God rewards only failure, not success.

We tripled our income over the next few years. Then I wrote three books and recorded lots of cassette albums and videocassette programs. A few years later, we were living on a golf course in Boca Raton, Florida. I was speaking full time, writing comedy, and living the dream.

What can happen when you open your mind to possibilities? What happens when you find your passion and let it run free?

Suddenly, and much to my astonishment, I wanted to look into my *own* windows at night and see the beautiful home and people wandering around talking to one another.

One weekend in 1981, we went to a movie, *The Continental Express*, starring the late John Belushi. This movie was loosely based on the career of Chicago *Tribune* journalist Mike Royko, who had always been a favorite of mine. Mike, I thought, had the life, writing for a famous newspaper and doing interviews on radio and TV. The next morning, I sent the editor of the *Boca Raton News* the following note:

> *Dear Wayne,*
>
> *I believe I can write as well as or better than anyone you have on staff. In order to prove that, I'd like to come to your office tomorrow morning at exactly ten o'clock. I'd like you to assign me two fresh topics of your choice. I will then have on your desk the next day two satire columns on those subjects. If anyone on your staff writes as well, tear them up. If they don't, I'm your new columnist.*

At ten the next morning, I was shown into his office. He assigned his two topics, and I wrote all night. A couple of weeks later, I was above the fold on the front page. Then, in true Royko fashion, I went down to the WSBR AM 740 radio station in Boca and asked to talk with the station manager. I told him I wanted my own radio show, and, after talking with me, he must have been thinking, *This guy?*

I do not have a radio voice, and my lisp makes me sound a bit effeminate. He took me into his office and said, "The price of an hour on our station is $2,000. If you can find sponsorship for an hour a week for thirteen weeks, you're in." The next day I tapped four friends to sponsor the show, telling them I'd make them famous by having them and their businesses featured on my shows.

When I returned to the radio station with four signed $500-a-week contracts for thirteen weeks, his jaw dropped. I sat alone in his office until the morning talent, Steve Haas, came in. He said something like, "I'm not sure how you sold those, but you and I have a ton of work to do if you're really going to have a show."

I showed up the next day for voice training with Steve.

"Okay, not bad," Steve said. "Try saying, 'It's sunny today' without whistling the 's' sound. And can you lower your voice this time, not your chin?"

After several grueling hours, I excused myself for a bathroom break. I was standing at the urinal when a very tall man walked up next to me, turned his head toward me, and said, "Hi. I haven't seen you here before."

I thought, *Oh, great. What's next?*

"Oh?" I said, staring straight ahead. "My name is Rick, and I'm taking speech therapy from Steve Haas."

"You're the guy who sold the thirteen weeks without knowing the price?"

"No, I knew the price," I said, defending myself. "It's $2,000 an hour."

He zipped up, stepped back, and looked right at me. "Our price for an hour on this little station is $500," he said. "Our guy didn't think you had a snowball's chance in hell at making those sales, so he inflated the price to get rid of you. I just fired him, and I'm giving you his job if you want it. You're now the general sales manager."

See the power of letting your passion run without restraint? The satire columnist and radio-show posts lasted about two years, and I continued professional speaking (doing corporate comedy) for another couple of years. Eventually I quit the speaking business due to travel. I could have quit traveling and started doing local seminars and coaching, but sometimes you get so close to the trees, you can't see the forest, you know? I decided to end my twenty-plus years of my Shaklee distributorship and start my own company selling, here's a shocker, vitamins. It's scary to risk a constant residual income that was difficult to develop. Plus, I did the math and figured that just my half of the distributorship would be paid over $500,000 in about twenty years (and it was). But it was a gamble I was willing to take. In 1995, Hillbrand Nutrition was born. I invested nearly half a million dollars of my own money into this venture. Two years after

I started it, I sold it to Alpine Industries, which later became EcoQuest, which then sold to Vollara. They wanted a speaker, and I wanted a break.

It was at Alpine that I learned the indoor air-quality business. On my own, I started researching patents to see what kind of technology might exist but had not yet made it to market. Six months later, I found an electron generator. Along with the advanced oxidation technology championed by the RGF Environmental Group, we designed a new product and received a patent.

Long story short, I took this new invention back to Shaklee's home office and sold them on the idea. In 1999, I was appointed Senior VP of sales.

Are you getting my drift? Are you thinking back to when I was standing on the beach in Tijuana, Mexico, unsure if I would live another week? At that moment I decided that instead of trying to regain my health, I would regain my life, change began to happen. There had to be a reason for me to eat all that green squishy stuff and drink awful things like wheatgrass juice. Do you need to hit the reset button today? Your life may depend on it.

AND I THOUGHT CANCER WAS BAD

Around 2003, I was on a Delta jet traveling from my home in Dallas to Pleasanton, California; at this point, I was heading the AirSource division at Shaklee. I was sitting up front and talking with a guy in the seat next to me. We were showing each other pictures of our families when he suddenly said, "We're very fortunate people, you and I. We have so much to be thankful for."

I nodded in response.

"And yet," he said, "none of us are more than thirty days away from being homeless and broke, given the right circumstances."

Whoa! Where did that come from? Here we were, having a little male-bonding session, and he dumps all over the party. I just looked at him for a few seconds before saying, "Look, I appreciate all that I have, but I have to disagree with your last comment. I *have* been blessed, but I also worked very hard for a long time to achieve whatever success I have. It's not up to fate or a couple of bad things happening. I've had my share of bad circumstances. How we respond to those is what defines us."

He looked at me, smiled, lifted his drink to toast mine, and said, "From your lips to God's ears." Clink.

To my shock and horror, in less than two years, I had lost my job, two houses, two cars, and I had filed for bankruptcy. Shaklee was up for sale, and the interim CEO was a magazine direct-sales guy who told me he wasn't renewing my contract, so I quit while I still had a job. I believed the old adage; "It's easier to get a job when you have one of those." Everyone who believes that, stand on your head.

I tried in vain to sell my homes but the market had already gone into the Dumpster and they were under water more than $100,000. Then the hurricanes hit South Florida and destroyed my condo. Stubbornly I just kept paying for everything until the money just ran out. I felt like I was in free-fall and all I could do when I hit the end of my rope was tie a knot and hold on. This had never happened to me before. I was always the go-to guy with all the answers. Hey, it's Rick—everything will be okay.

Losing everything was every bit as hard and challenging as having cancer. Having a car repossessed in front of your neighbors is a memorable event. "Wow, Rick," a neighbor said, "you're one important guy. When you call AAA for a tow, they send the sheriff too."

Having a judge ask you if you have any more jewelry to declare is humbling. Living in your ex-wife's basement and borrowing a car from your son is where your butt hits the ground. Depression sets in, and your immune system craps out. I ran up an $8,000 hospital bill with simple bronchitis. I was starting to read the obituary columns daily to set new goals.

What kept me from jumping off a bridge is that I had already been nearly fatal once. I had already fought for my life and won. I'd already established my passion, but I'd made an error. I'd put the future of that passion into someone else's care. Someone else had control over my life. But my family was there for me, including my kids, my brother, and Barbara, my ex-wife. They loaned or gave me money and it kept me from being homeless. And then one morning I woke up early and remembered my conversation with that guy on the Delta flight.

And yet none of us are more than thirty days away from being homeless and broke, given the right circumstances.

It was time for me to hit the reset button for the second time.

There is always time. I'm pulling for you, because I've been in the jaws of death twice now. And I'm here to tell you not to focus on getting well or getting rich. Focus on living the life that God *specifically* gave to you and not to someone else. President Kennedy was asked what the definition of success was and he responded, "The ancient Greek definition of happiness was the full use of your powers for success."

It's time for you and me to join hands and walk forward into the future that's waiting to see what we can do. You will survive simply because someone else's future and your future are connected. In short, it matters to me and everyone else if you live or die.

Let me bring to an end our time together with the little mouse, Reepicheep, from C. S. Lewis's books, *The Chronicles of Narnia*. When the mythical ship, *The Dawn Treader*, had entered dark, unfamiliar waters, much like the ones you may be facing now, the crew decided not to go farther. Reepicheep, the brave little mouse, wanted to continue the mission. Captain Drinian, one of the protagonists, asked Reepicheep heatedly, "What manner of use would it be plowing through that blackness?"

"Use?" replied Reepicheep. "Use, Captain? . . . So far as I know we did not set sail for things useful but to seek honor and adventures."

For your free copy of Rick's report,
Ten Strategies for Long-Term Survival after Cancer,
Log on to http://www.freespeakersgroup.com and leave your name and e-mail address.